How To Be A Better Wife

By

Mary Franklin.C.

THANK YOU, PAGE

Greetings, Readers. I appreciate your decision to embark on the journey of being a more devoted wife. I applaud your commitment to personal growth and relationship improvement, as it is evident in your willingness to research this topic and strengthen your marriage.

You've taken the initial step in creating a more solid and fulfilling marriage by arriving at this book and browsing through the content. It shows that you are committed to investing in and giving priority to the success of your relationship that you want to learn and develop in this area of your life.

I want you to connect with the material in this book, think critically about its insights, and apply its ideas to your relationships and life. Every chapter has been thoughtfully crafted to offer you ideas and suggestions for strengthening your position as a wife and developing a lasting relationship with your partner.

Please share your ideas and experiences by leaving a review once you've finished the book. Your feedback is extremely important to me as an author and will also assist other readers in making well-informed decisions about how this book will benefit them in their journey towards a happier marriage.

Keep in mind that growing as a wife is a lifelong journey of self-awareness, development, and love. It requires persistence, open communication, and a willingness to grow from both successes and setbacks. Seize the chance to deepen and broaden your relationship, and never undervalue the transformative power of little, deliberate actions in creating a lasting marriage.

Again, I want to thank you for opening this book and reading its pages. I hope it helps, directs, and uplifts you as you strive to be the greatest wife you can be. Warm regards. [Mary Franklin. C.].

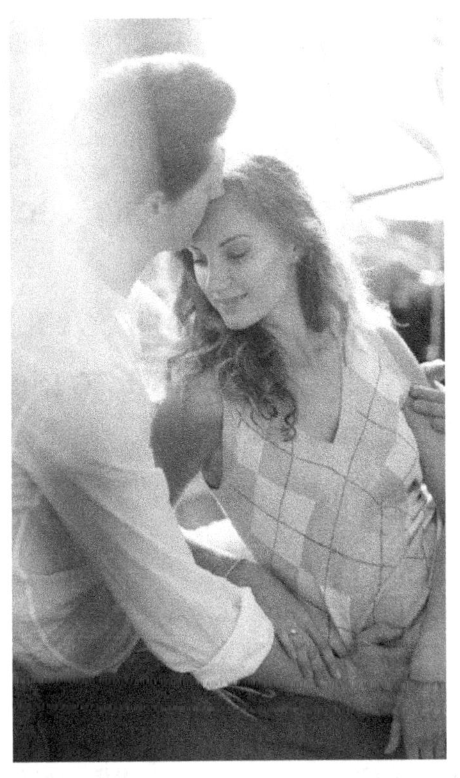

TABLE OF CONTENTS

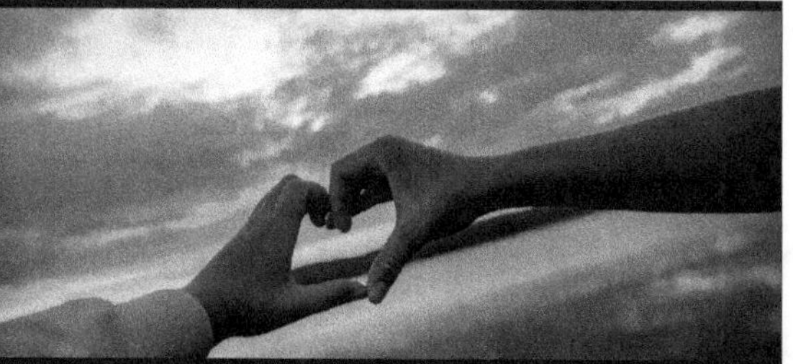

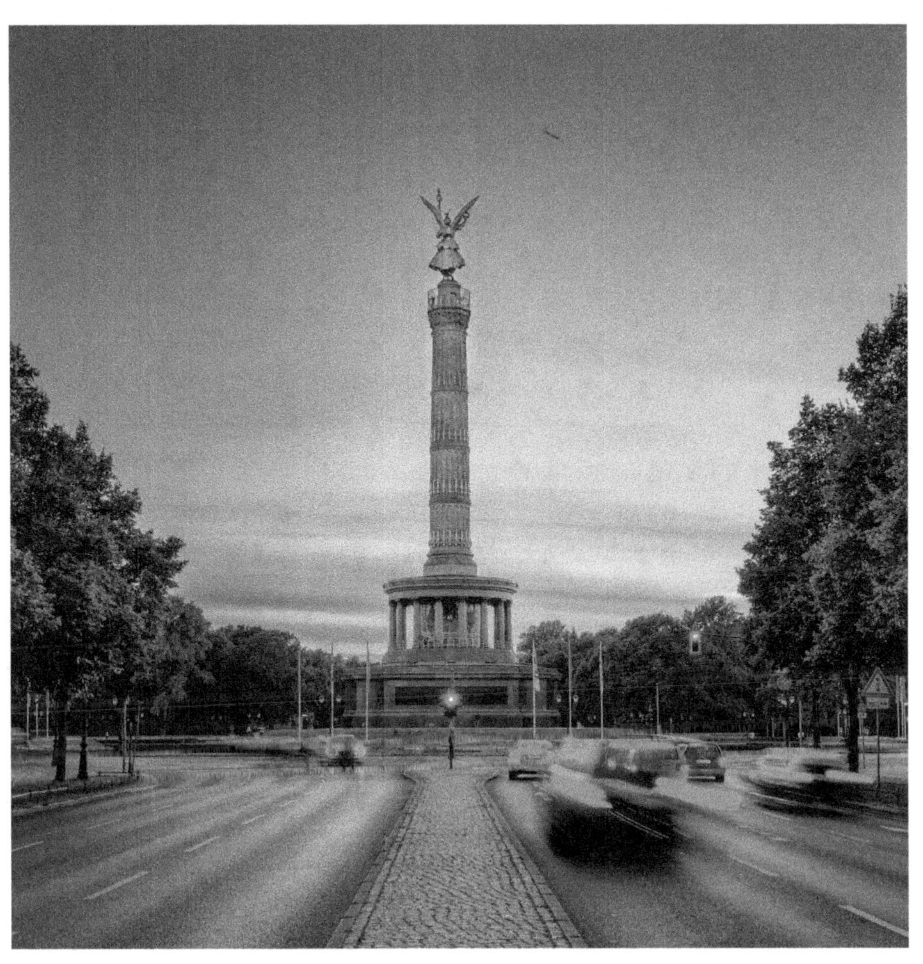

Become The Pillar Of Your Home.

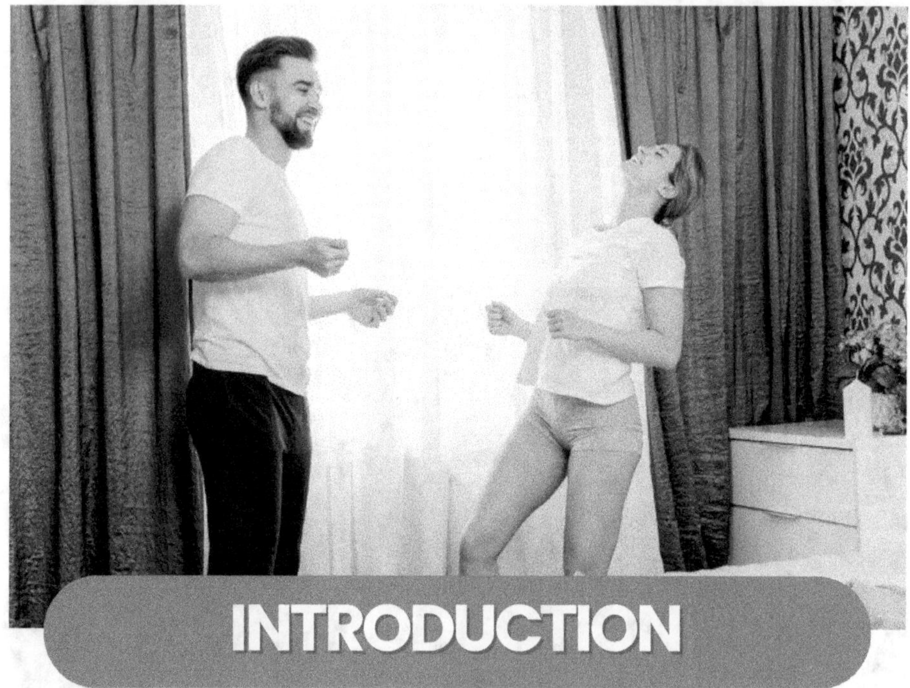

INTRODUCTION

Once upon a time, in a small hamlet set amid rolling hills and lush vegetation, there lived a woman named Mary Franklin C. Mary was well-known across the community for her pleasant smile, calm manner, and strong commitment to her family.

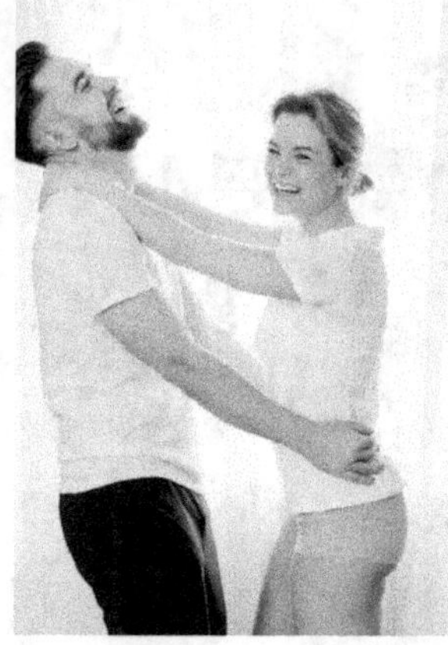

Mary committed herself when she married her beloved husband, Clinton, to always prioritize and nurture their relationship. She saw that establishing a long-term marriage took more than simply love; it also required dedication, communication, and consistent work.

Mary understood that caring for her husband and children was more than a duty; it was a privilege. She approached each day with a strategy, making certain that her family's needs were addressed with love and attention. She diligently planned their schedules, cooked nutritious meals, and provided a comfortable home environment.

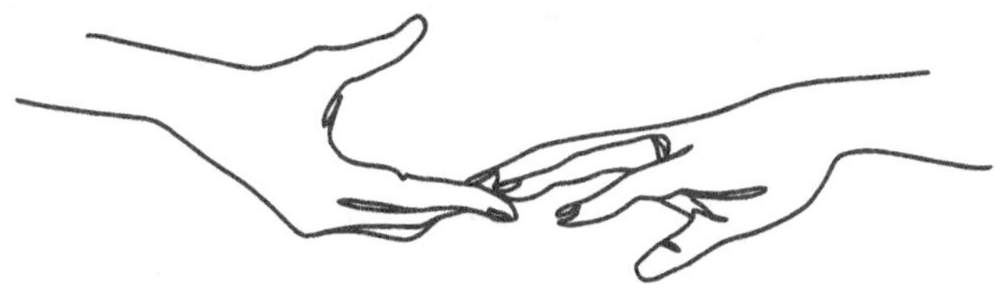

But Mary's preparations went beyond just practicalities. She recognized the value of emotional support and connection in sustaining a healthy family link. She made it a point to spend meaningful time with her husband and children, whether through shared meals, family vacations, or heartfelt chats by the fireside. Mary stressed honesty and perseverance in her quest for her family's long-term happiness.

She believed that open and honest communication was essential for a good relationship, and she encouraged her family to express themselves freely and without fear of judgment. Mary was a source of strength for her family in both happy and difficult times. She met each challenge with grace and courage, relying on her unfailing confidence in the power of love to get her through.

And, certainly, Mary's passion and affection resulted in her family's happiness and peace. Their home was filled with laughter, joy, and the obvious warmth of a love that recognized no boundaries. They faced life's twists and turns together, reinforced by their unshakeable loyalty to one another.

As Mary gazed around at her husband and children, she couldn't help but be overwhelmed with gratitude. She understood that their love was a gift, one that she would treasure and cultivate for the rest of her life. And so, in the embrace of her cherished family, Mary discovered her greatest joy—the simple yet profound delight that comes from living a life filled with love, honesty, dedication, and everlasting bliss.

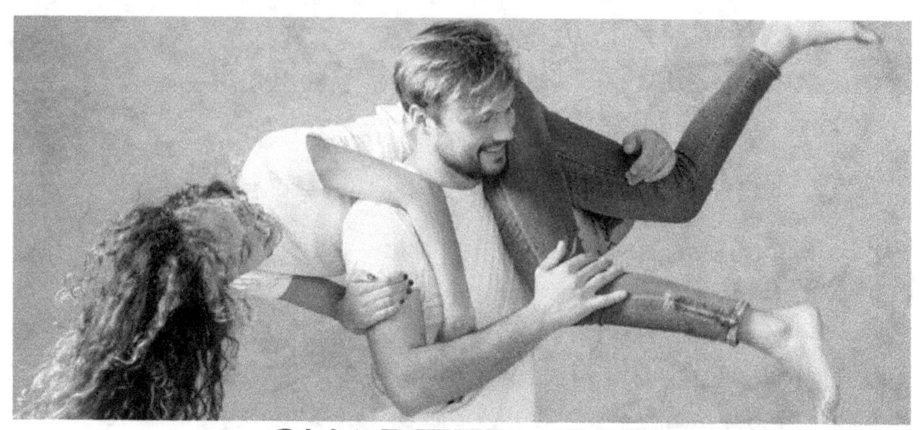

CHAPTER ONE

THE IMPORTANCE OF BEING A BETTER WIFE

Being a more loving wife means growing your affection and bond with your lover, resulting in a link that grows deeper every day. Little deeds of generosity, tender words, and enjoyable time spent together enhance a bond characterized by warmth, understanding, and profound emotional closeness.

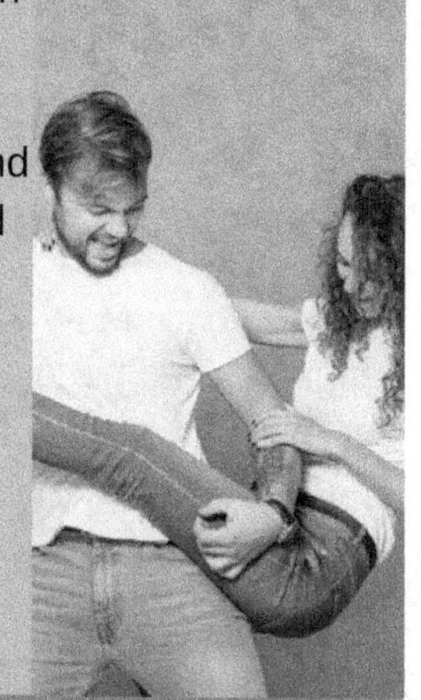

As you prioritize your union and invest in its development, you will discover that your devotion for each other develops into something genuinely beautiful and enduring, complementing your life in ways you didn't know were imaginable.

Being a better wife is more than just a role; it's a commitment to nurturing your relationship and building a strong foundation for a lasting marriage. Here's why it matters:

1. Building up Emotional Connectivity

Let's explore how to improve feeling connectivity in marriages. Imagine your romantic bond as a fragile flower that needs attention and care to thrive.

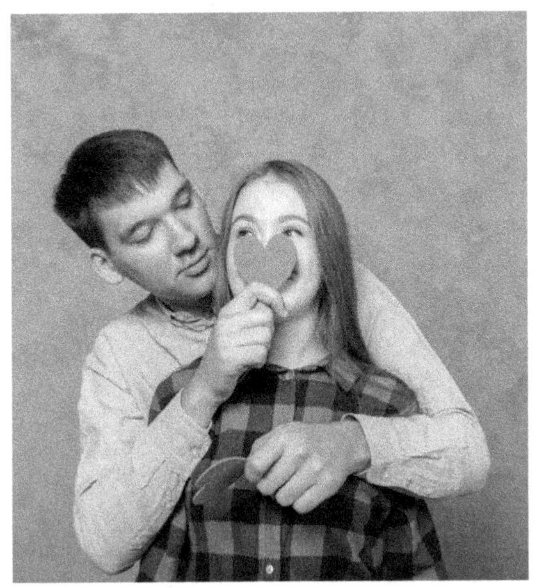

I've witnessed the enormous power of an intense sense of emotion in a couple's relationship. So let's look at this together in a manner that's interesting, relatable, and understandable. First, allow me to put together an illustration for you using facts from my own life.

Imagine a regular evening at home with the person I love, Clinton. We're sitting on the couch together, telling stories about our day, laughing at ridiculous jokes, and holding hands while watching our favourite movie. In those moments, I can feel the comforting presence of our emotional connection wrap over us like a cosy blanket, encompassing us in an understanding of tenderness, confidence, and closeness.

Now, let's look at what it means to strengthen emotional connections. It's more than just spending time together; it's about actually bonding on a deeper level and openly discussing your ideas, feelings, and dreams. It's about being there and sensitive to your partner's needs, relating with compassion and comprehension, and providing assistance and support in both good and terrible situations.

Consider feelings of attachment as the glue that maintains the connections between you and your lover together. When you focus on strengthening this relationship, you lay a solid basis for your marriage's success. You develop an aura of reliability and safety that allows you to face every obstacle in life together, knowing that you constantly have each other's backs.

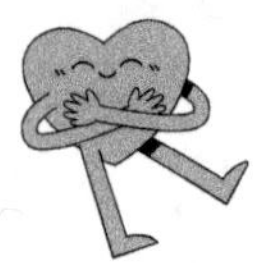

But how do you strengthen emotional connections? It's all about making deliberate attempts that should take precedence over your relationship while enjoying quality time together. Every small gesture matters, whether it's through regular date nights, passionate chats, or simple gestures of compassion and affection. For example, my husband Clinton and I schedule a weekly "check-in" to discuss our thoughts, aspirations, and plans.

This focused time allows us to be connected and in tune with each other's wants and desires, building our bond in the process. A successful and fulfilling marriage requires a strong feeling. By fostering this connection with love, care, and thoughtfulness, you create a long-lasting relationship—one filled with love, trust, and joy that becomes deeper and stronger with each passing day.

2. Growing Trust and Mutual Respect:

Trust and shared dignity operate as the cornerstone of a strong marriage. Without them, the structure will disintegrate; with them, your connection with one another will be able to resist everything life throws at it.

Imagine this scenario: You and your partner are arranging a weekend away. The air is filled with eagerness and expectation as you pack your luggage and make arrangements. You know your spouse will keep their vows, be there for you when you need them, and always have your greatest goals in mind.

So, how can you foster tolerance and respect for one another in your connection with one another? It begins with straightforward interaction and honesty. Share your views, thoughts, and worries with your partner, and listen to them in turn.

Be open about your goals, and always follow through on your promises. For example, my husband, Clinton, and I have a rule in our marriage: no secrets. We make a point of communicating honestly and openly with one another, even when it is challenging. This has built a solid basis of trust amongst us, as we know we can always count on one another to be open and clear.

A further vital component is respecting each other's limits and independence. Honour your partner's uniqueness, opinions, and choices, even if they are different from yours. Celebrate each other's abilities and help each other grow and develop.
We make it a point in our marriage to verify each other's feelings and viewpoints, even if we do not always agree. By demonstrating understanding and sympathy, we build our link and increase mutual respect.

Finally, this is a continuous process that involves effort, patience, and attention from both partners. However, the advantages are tremendous. With confidence and respect for each other at the core of your marriage, you can withstand any storm and rise happier and healthier than before.

3. Promoting Intimacy and Romance:

Picture this: You and your lover are snuggled up on the couch, basking in the soft glow of candlelight, exchanging romantic whispers and stolen kisses. There's a spark in the air, a magical feeling that fires your hearts and spirits, bringing you more closely with each passing moment.

But how can you grow closeness and romanticism in your marriage? It's all about generating periods of closeness and passion to keep the fires of love burning strong. Intimacy refers to the strong feelings you enjoy with your companion, whilst romanticism adds an added layer of excitement and attraction.

Let me explain this concept with a story from my marriage to Clinton. Clinton surprised me one evening with a home-cooked dinner under the stars. As we sat together, savouring each exquisite bite and taking in the grandeur of the night sky, I felt a sense of feeling of being connected that made my heart sing.

Now, let's look at some practical techniques to increase nearness and dedication in your relationship:

1. Value Quality Time:

Set aside a particular period for yourself with the one you love, free of distractions and obligations. Whether it's a romantic dinner date, a cosy movie night at home, or a stroll hand in hand, treasure these moments together.

2. Speak Plainly and Sincerely:

Express your views, feelings, and desires to your spouse, and urge them to do the same. Open communication fosters trust and improves emotional connections, establishing a foundation for tenderness and love to thrive.

3. Express Affection Openly:

Don't be scared to convey how much you care for your mate with simple acts of generosity and tenderness. Let your lover know how much you care about them, whether through a charming love letter tucked into their lunchbox or a delicate caress as you pass by.

4. Keep your Love Alive:

Make your love life more exciting by trying new things and going on trips together. Try new activities, and explore different types of closeness while maintaining your hunger alive in your marriage.

5. Surprise and Delight:

Tell your lover how much you care through nice acts and performing acts of kindness for them. Allow your creativity and spontaneity to flourish, whether you're planning an unexpected date night or putting love notes throughout the house.

By cultivating closeness and romance in your union, you set up a genuinely amazing love story—one brimming with times of happiness, enthusiasm, and closeness that you will cherish forever. So, dearest friend, relish the beauty of love and let your hearts dance to the rhythm of passion.

4. Establishing a Harmonious Family Environment:

Let's look into the excellent concept of designing a happy household atmosphere. Picture this: You and your family sat around the banquet table, laughing, telling stories, and eating excellent food. The air is filled with warmth and unity, a sense of feeling of belonging that makes your heart sing.

But how do you foster such an enjoyable family setting? It's all about instilling respect, affection, and comprehension among family members and setting up an atmosphere in which everybody feels appreciated, supported, and loved.

Let me demonstrate this point with a personal experience from my family. One weekend, we decided to hold a family game night. We gathered around the table, everyone bringing our favourite board games and refreshments, and the excitement in the air was apparent. Throughout the evening, we joked, mocked, and encouraged each other, making memories that would last a lifetime.

Now, let's go over some practical techniques to establish a happy family environment:

1. Support open and honest conversation amongst relatives.

Set up a secure atmosphere in which anyone may share their views, emotions, and worries without worrying about criticism or judgment.

2. Set up Boundaries:

Set up explicit limits and standards within the family. Honour each other's private areas and confidentiality, and establish standards that foster genuine kindness and consideration for each other.

3. Resolve Conflict Peacefully:

Controversy is an unavoidable aspect of familial relationships, but it is critical to deal with it effectively and productively. Teach your kids how to handle problems calmly, listen to each other's viewpoints, and create solutions that benefit everyone involved.

4. Express Appreciation:

Take the time to acknowledge each other's accomplishments and efforts within the family. Whether it's a simple thank you or a passionate comment, expressing gratitude promotes happiness and friendliness among family members.

Creating a happy family environment fosters a sense of unity and belonging, which enhances the family link and brings you closer together. So, my dear friend, embrace the beauty of family and make your home full of love, laughter, and pleasure.

5. Supporting personal growth and fulfilment:

Let's discuss the enriching topic of promoting personal growth and contentment inside your marriage. Picture this: You and the one you love sit side by side, encouraging each other as you achieve your hopes and goals.

It's a source of pleasure and satisfaction to see each other succeed, knowing that you're both there to promote and promote each other every step of the way. But how can you foster my development and fulfilment within your relationship? It's about establishing a space in which both partners feel encouraged to follow what they love to do, investigate their passions, and realize their full potential.

Let me demonstrate this concept with a tale from my relationship. When I indicated a desire to complete my studies and pursue a job as a relationship therapist, my husband, Clinton, was my strongest supporter.

He inspired me to pursue my aspirations, helped me overcome obstacles, and celebrated my accomplishments alongside me every step of the way.

Now, let's go over some practical techniques to support yourself and find happiness in your romantic life:

1. Promote Each Other's Goals:

Listen to your partner's targets, visions, and achievements and provide unflinching support and encouragement. Whether they are exploring a new professional route, adopting a hobby, or going on a way to grow personally journey, be there to encourage them and provide direction and support throughout the way.

2. Foster a Growth-Focused Environment:

Create a culture of growth and learning in your relationship, encouraging both partners to move outside of their comfort zones and embrace new chances for personal improvement. Share materials, attend workshops or seminars together, and go on learning excursions as a group.

3. Celebrate Each Other's Successes:

Take time to acknowledge one another for victories, no matter how big or small. Whether it's getting a new job, learning a new skill, or reaching a personal milestone, acknowledge and celebrate one another's accomplishments with real enthusiasm and joy.

4. Offer Emotional Support:

Be there for your partner when facing the inevitable obstacles and failures that come with personal growth and development.

Offer a listening ear, words of encouragement, and a shoulder to lean on when things become tough, knowing that you'll be there for each other through thick and thin.

5. Grow Together:
As a partnership, accept one another by setting shared objectives, doing new things jointly, and pushing one another to be the greatest versions of yourselves. Growing and adapting together strengthens your link and fosters a long-lasting partnership.

Nurturing personal growth and fulfilment in your marriage fosters an exciting and healthy connection in which both individuals can attain all of their abilities and live their best lives. So, my dear buddy, accept the journey of discovering yourself together and watch your relationship thrive and expand in beautiful ways.

Plans for Being a Better Wife:

1. Show Appreciation and Affection Daily:

Showing praise and affection daily is like filling your partnership's love tank. It maintains the affection alive and broadens what you share with your companion.
Furthermore, it's a terrific method of reiterating to one another why you were in love the first time. So, take a moment every day to express how much you love and adore your partner. Small gestures, such as a meaningful compliment, a warm embrace, or a simple "I love you," can have a major effect on your relationship.

2. Support Each Other's Goals and Dreams:

Let's discuss how to encourage one other's goals and hopes in your relationship. It's like feeling each other's biggest cheerleader, rooting for your spouse to succeed and realize their objectives. For example, suppose you want to establish your firm and your partner supports and encourages you every step of the way. They help you explore ideas, assist you with duties, and commemorate your accomplishments with you.

Supporting one another's desire to succeed entails being able to serve each other no matter what. It's about believing in your partner's potential and doing whatever you can to assist them achieve their goals.

Take the time to listen to your lover's dreams and aspirations, and provide constant support and encouragement. Be there for your spouse, whether it's by listening, offering guidance, or providing practical assistance. Show them that you adhere to them and their aspirations. Together, you are capable of doing anything you set yourself up to.

3. Prioritize Self-Care and Well-Being:

Let's talk about the value of emphasizing taking care of oneself and wellness in your marriage. It's similar to putting on a respirator first before aiding others on a plane: you must take good care of yourself before you can care for others.

Consider self-care to be taking the time to replenish your batteries and improve the state of your body, mind, and emotions. It is about acting in pursuits that make you sensational, at ease, and fulfilled. Let's say both you and your lover agree to highlight personal care together. You go for walks in nature, try meditation or mindfulness, or simply relax at home with an excellent book or movie. Individual self-care enables you to be your most effective self in your marriage.

Setting aside taking care of oneself and wellness is not selfish; it is necessary for a successful and fulfilling relationship. When you take time to look after yourself, you'll be more capable of showing up for your lover and helping them on their wellness path.

Setting aside taking care of oneself and wellness is not selfish; it is necessary for a successful and fulfilling relationship. When you take time to look after yourself, you'll be more capable of showing up for your lover and helping them on their wellness path.

Consider personal care a top concern in your romantic life. Make a habit of spending time with yourself, whether it's for a workout, relaxation, or passion, and urge your lover to follow suit. Keep in mind that a happy marriage starts by taking custody of yourself first.

Personal Experience:

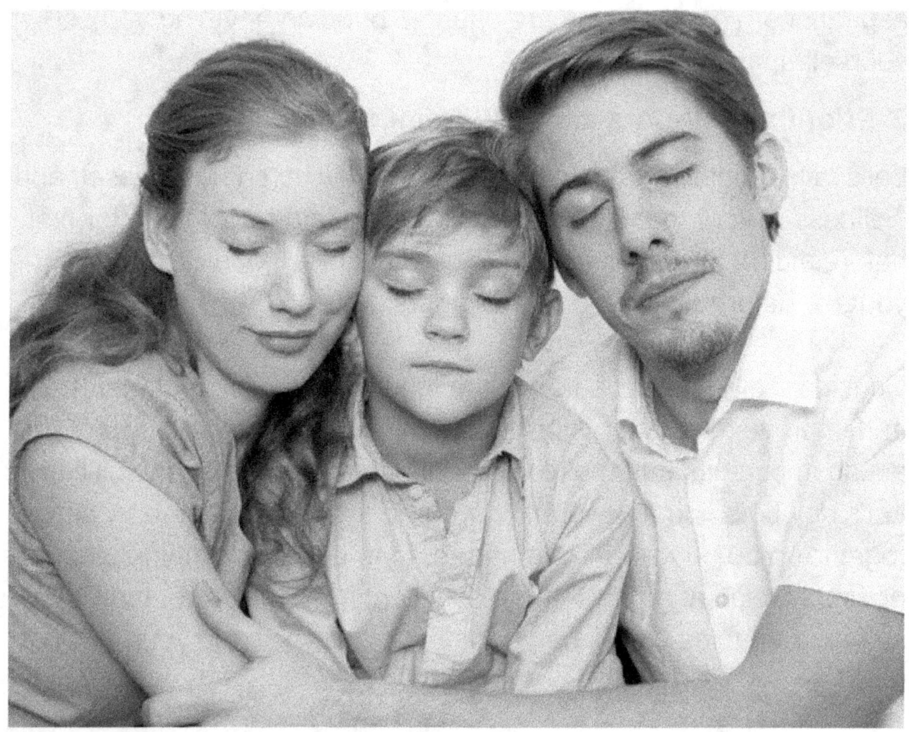

Being a better wife has positively impacted my marriage with my husband, Clinton. By putting our relationship first, engaging in communication and closeness, and believing in each other's aspirations and dreams, we've built a strong and loving connection that brings us joy and fulfilment every day.

Through our journey together, I've realized that being a better wife is about more than just making my husband happy; it's about cultivating our relationship and building a foundation of love, trust, and mutual respect that will carry us through life's ups and downs.

So, as you continue on your road to becoming a better wife, keep in mind the value of deepening emotional connections, establishing trust and respect, encouraging intimacy and love, creating an enjoyable family atmosphere, and promoting personal development and happiness. Setting goals for these qualities can not only enhance your marriage but also provide you with an added feeling of love and enjoyment.

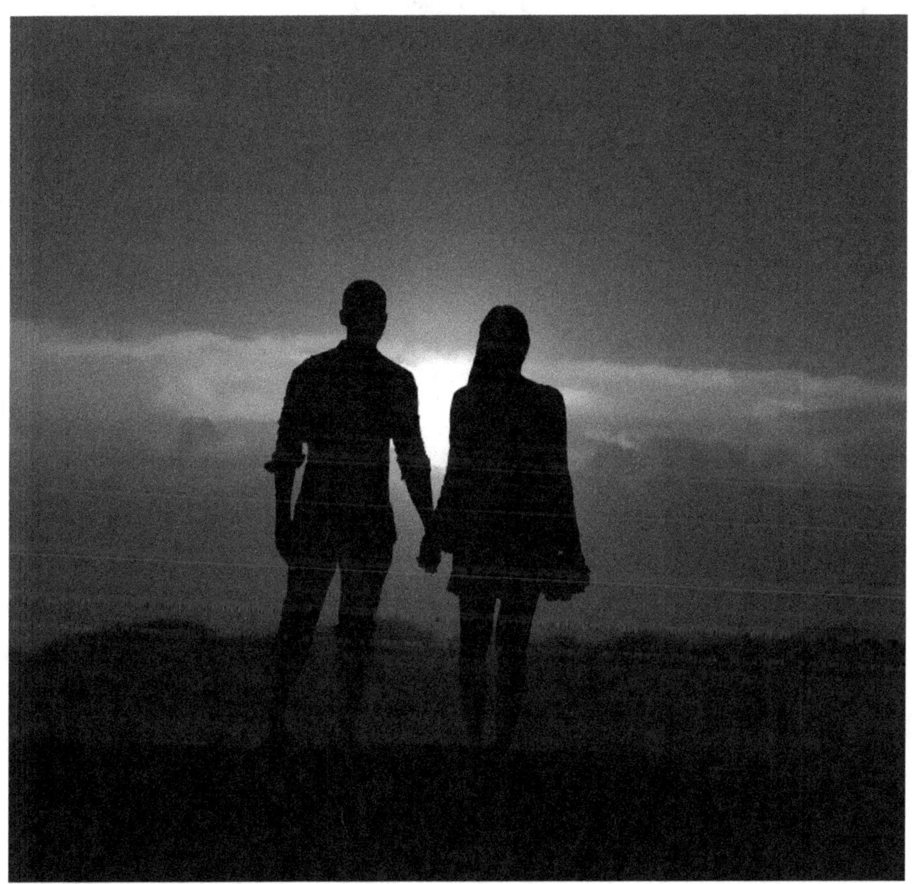

CHAPTER TWO
WHAT IS YOUR ROLE AS WIFE?

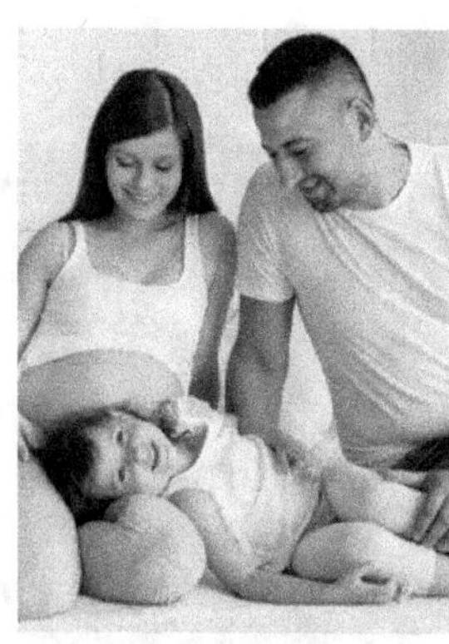

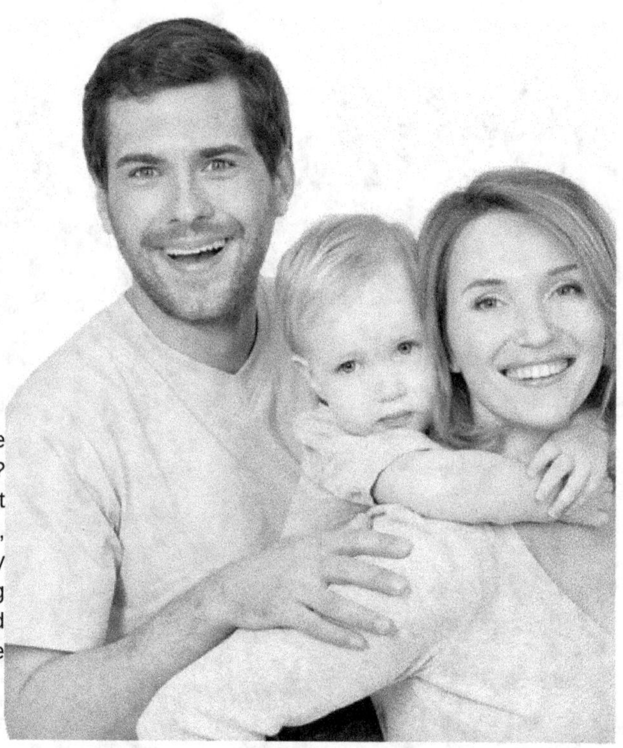

Hey there, how about we discuss the role of a wife? Now, I understand that it might be challenging at times, but believe me when I say that it is all about accepting your unique journey and finding joy in the simple moments.

So, what does it mean to be a wife?

Consider the tastes of yourself to be your family's heart—the person who ties everything together with love, care, and kindness. Your duty is more than just about cooking meals and doing laundry (though those things are important too!), it's about being a partner, a confidante, and a source of strength for your husband.

I recall the first time I was married to Clinton Franklin. I was happy, anxious, and not sure what it meant to be a wife. But as time passed, I realized that being a wife is a precious tie based on trust, respect, and unshakable love—it's much more than just a title.

Undoubtedly more than at any other moment in history, women today want a clear grasp of how they should interact with their partners. The tremendous changes in society brought about by the women's liberation movement over the previous few decades have caused so much uncertainty that the very concept of "roles" offends certain individuals. They believe that adhering to an "outdated standard" will cause them to lose their distinctive qualities and independence.

It's critical to carefully examine the Bible's teachings on the topic at hand. And, while the Word of God does not use what is now known as a "role" to describe marriage, it is explicit about the specific tasks that God gives to a wife.

1. Let's talk about the necessity of being an aid to your husband, and I'll use an example from my own life to demonstrate this concept.

As a relationship therapist, I've witnessed firsthand the importance of connection and support in marriage. Being a helper to your man is more than just accomplishing duties or meeting his wants; it is also about being his ally, cheerleader, and partner in every meaning of the word.

According to Genesis, God made Eve to be a fitting helper for Adam. Although the word "helper" seems straightforward, Its meaning is complex. "Ezer," which means "helper" in original Hebrew, is a word that the Bible uses to refer to God as our helper. This demonstrates the importance of a wife's assistance role to her husband—it is a position of power, encouragement, and divine purpose.

Let me now tell you a story about my marriage to Clinton. My husband Clinton Franklin was pursuing a job shift early in our relationship, which took a lot of time, energy, and commitment. Seeing his enthusiasm for this new route as his wife, I realized it was my duty to help him in every way I could.

I took on more household chores so he could devote more time to his work and study. When he encountered difficulties or failures, I gave him words of support and reminded him of his value. Above all, I supported him, never faltering in my faith in his potential and his aspirations. My husband helped me out in return, encouraging me to follow my passions and professional ambitions.

We developed into one another's biggest supporters, encouraging and assisting one another in reaching our full potential.
I discovered from this experience that supporting one another involves more than simply what you do; it also involves the attitude and perspective you bring to your union. It involves treating one another with respect, love, and an eagerness to go above and above to support them.

Therefore, my dear friend, keep in mind the ability you have to support your man as you walk your journey as a woman.
Accept this position with open arms, knowing that your encouragement and support will enable him to realize his full potential and soar to new heights. Who knows? Along the way, you could discover that supporting your partner strengthens your relationship and infuses love, pleasure, and purpose into your marriage.

2. Let's discuss the value of showing him respect and how it could boost your union.

Paul stresses the value of wives obeying their husbands in Ephesians 5:33. However, what exactly would it imply to honour the love of one's life? It's not enough just to accept his existence; you also need to treat him with deference and honour him in every area of your connection with each other.

Let me now use a story from my marriage to Clinton Franklin to explain this idea. Clinton felt defeated one evening when he got home from work. He wanted someone to listen to him, to encourage him, and to cheer him up after a trying day at work.

I listened to him with respect and compassion rather than downplaying his experiences or ignoring his sentiments. I gave him confidence in his abilities, acknowledged his feelings, and reminded him of all the things I valued and liked in him.
Clinton's behaviour changed during the evening, and I could see it. The knowledge that he had a partner who genuinely believed in him and backed him without reservation made him stand a little taller and smile a little brighter.
Showing your husband respect also entails attending to his needs. Each man needs something different, be it companionship, self-assurance, or just a sense of a need. You can communicate to your husband that you appreciate him and are concerned about his well-being by paying attention to his needs and making an effort to address them.
My husband and I put respect for one another's wants and preferences first in our marriage. We always try to aid one another, both in good and difficult times, and we speak honestly and frankly with one another. We pay attention to each other with empathy.
I hope you will keep in mind the importance of respect in your marriage as you sail your journey as a wife, my dear buddy. You're building a firm basis of love, trust, and enduring gratitude for the one you love when you acknowledge and value him. You're also improving how you relate as a pair.

3. Let's talk more about the value of loving one another and how it might improve your marriage. Let's discuss this together.

As a relationship therapist, I have personally seen the transformative power of love in a marriage.
Titus 2:4 exhorts wives to love their husbands. However, what does loving your husband mean? It is more than just love or warmth; it is accepting him for who he is, imperfections and all.

It's about deciding to create a meaningful and close bond with him, appreciating him for who he is, and realizing his value.

Love, for both my husband Clinton and me, is the cornerstone of our union. It is what keeps us going through life's highs and lows, pleasures and difficulties. We now know that love is more than simply an emotion; it's a decision to put each other's well-being and joy first.

The closeness of a relationship is a crucial yet frequently disregarded component of love. Surveys, as you indicated, indicate that one of a man's primary demands is sex. In addition to strengthening their physical bond, wives who actively participate in a fulfilling sexual relationship with their husbands also increase their emotional bond.

Clinton and I place a high value on intimacy in our marriage and routinely take care of our physical bond. We work to establish a secure and loving environment where we can freely explore and express our love for each other, and we communicate openly about our wants and desires.

However, love is more than just having sex; it's about letting your man know that you cherish and value him in every area of your life together. The goal is to help him feel heard, seen, and understood despite the distractions and busyness of daily life.

To me, showing Clinton that he is always in my thoughts and my heart is a sign of love. Every day I try to make him feel loved and appreciated, whether it's by little acts of kindness, considerate deeds of service, or just spending time listening to him with compassion and empathy.

Therefore, my dear friend, keep in mind that love is a decision—a daily commitment to put your relationship first and strengthen your bond—as you travel the path of loving your husband. Accepting love in all its manifestations will improve your marriage and lay the groundwork for a lifetime of closeness, trust, and happiness.

4. Let's clarify the commonly misinterpreted idea of surrendering to your husband's leadership.

Being a relationship therapist, I've come across a lot of myths about this subject, so let's talk about them collectively.
Both men and women may experience intense feelings and reactions when they hear the word "submission." Some people might think it's an outdated idea that implies women are less valuable than males or that they have to give up their individuality and independence. Others worry that if they submit, their husbands will abuse or dominate them.

But let's examine submission more closely, specifically as it relates to matrimony. As the church is based on Christ, so too are wives to submit to their partners.

"Wives, surrender to the men in your life just as you'd do to the Almighty. Because Jesus is the supreme leader of the church and likewise the body's Savior, the husband is the leader of the wife. However, just as the Christian community is under Christ, wives ought to give in to their partners in all matters.

Husbands, cherish your wives as much as Christ did, as He bestowed upon His life for the church to purify her after cleansing her with the word. This would allow Him to reveal the religious services to Himself in all her beauty, without a single stain, pucker up, or imperfection.

Consequently, men should love their wives as much as they care for their selves. Since no person has ever despised their flesh, but rather nurtures and protects it, as Jesus does with his followers since we are a part of His body, he who adores his wife also loves himself." Ephesians 5:22–30 reminds us.

However, what does this entail in real life? Giving in to your husband's every whim or mindlessly following his orders is not what submission is all about.

Rather, the focus should be on acknowledging and valuing his leadership role within the marriage. It's about keeping your agency and voice in the relationship but still accepting and trusting his decisions.

It has been a journey of respect, cooperation, and communication on my part to submit to my husband Clinton's leadership. It's about acknowledging his skills and putting my faith in his discernment, all the while being honest and forthright in my expression of my ideas. Clinton and I had to make a big financial decision at one point, as I recall. Even though we didn't agree on the best course of action, we listened to each other's viewpoints and eventually concluded jointly, with Clinton taking the lead because of his knowledge of the subject.

It doesn't mean that I lose my identity or turn into a helpless spectator in our marriage when I submit to Clinton's leadership. Rather, the focus should be on collaborating as equal partners, where each of us contributes our distinct abilities and viewpoints. It's critical to remember that submitting requires reciprocity. Women must submit to their husbands, and men must love their wives selflessly, as Christ loved the church. This entails prioritizing your spouse's needs over your own, loving and caring for them, and making an effort to strengthen and assist them in all facets of life.

So, my friend, please keep in mind that honouring and appreciating the distinct duties that you share in your union defines what requires you to negotiate the idea of submitting to your husband's leadership rather than giving up your independence or power. In addition to fortifying your relationship with your partner, you will lay the groundwork for enduring trust, love, and honour by accepting submission in a sensible and balanced manner.

5. Assisting my husband in achieving all that the LORD has for him.

These verses make it quite evident that a wife must willingly submit to her husband's kind and kind guidance. I am therefore fulfilling my husband as I willingly surrender to him. I'm assisting him in carrying out his obligations and shaping him into the husband, man, and leader that God designed him to be. The finest couples are those in which both partners agree to carry out their duties willingly and without duress.

For Clinton to fulfil his divine role as a servant leader, he requires my kind regard and cooperation. And I find it easier to submit to Clinton's leadership when he loves me in the manner that he is led to. I approach this with a mindset of giving myself over to God.

Peter wrote in one of his letters that despite Jesus's excruciating suffering and insults, He "kept committing Himself to Him who judges righteously" instead of taking revenge (1 Peter 2:23). Being the wife of a flawed guy is much easier when you give your life to the Father, especially if you may have arguments.

An important note: Some of you might be living abusive lives or in extremely toxic and disastrous marriage environments. It could occasionally be improper or even dangerous for you to implement the submitting principles blindly.

For instance, you should take action to safeguard your children and yourself if you are experiencing verbal or physical abuse. If that describes you, please seek sensible counsel from your therapist or another qualified someone to assist you with your particular problem. It is not necessary to become a doormat or to put up with seriously harmful behaviour indefinitely to be loving, forgiving, and obedient.

How everything works together.

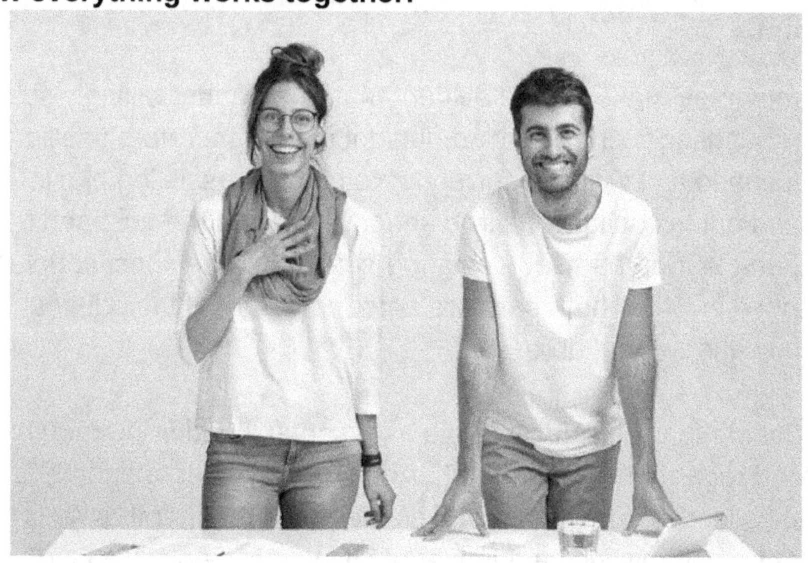

You are familiar with how a pattern functions if you have ever attempted to sew or finish a dress. Numerous small and large components make up the design, and none of them truly resemble the final product. After laying out the pattern and cutting the fabric, all you have are some fabric scraps instead of an actual outfit.

Together, these parts form a full garment when fastened together correctly and finished with buttons, snaps, or a zipper. All patterns consist of pairs of parts: there are two pieces for the sleeves, two pieces for the bodice, a front and back skirt, and even the collar and facing are typically in pairs. Marriage is a lot like that.

God has created a master blueprint for women and husbands that, when followed, will result in a complete, functional, and lovely marriage. My marriage might not look the same as yours, just as a garment can be created in a range of colours and sizes with countless variations in detail from one pattern.
We must resolve our marital issues by God's design as we confess Christ as the Lord of our lives. Every wife needs to realize her role, adhere to God's plan, and make an effort to fulfil her husband's obligations.

Accepting Your Path.

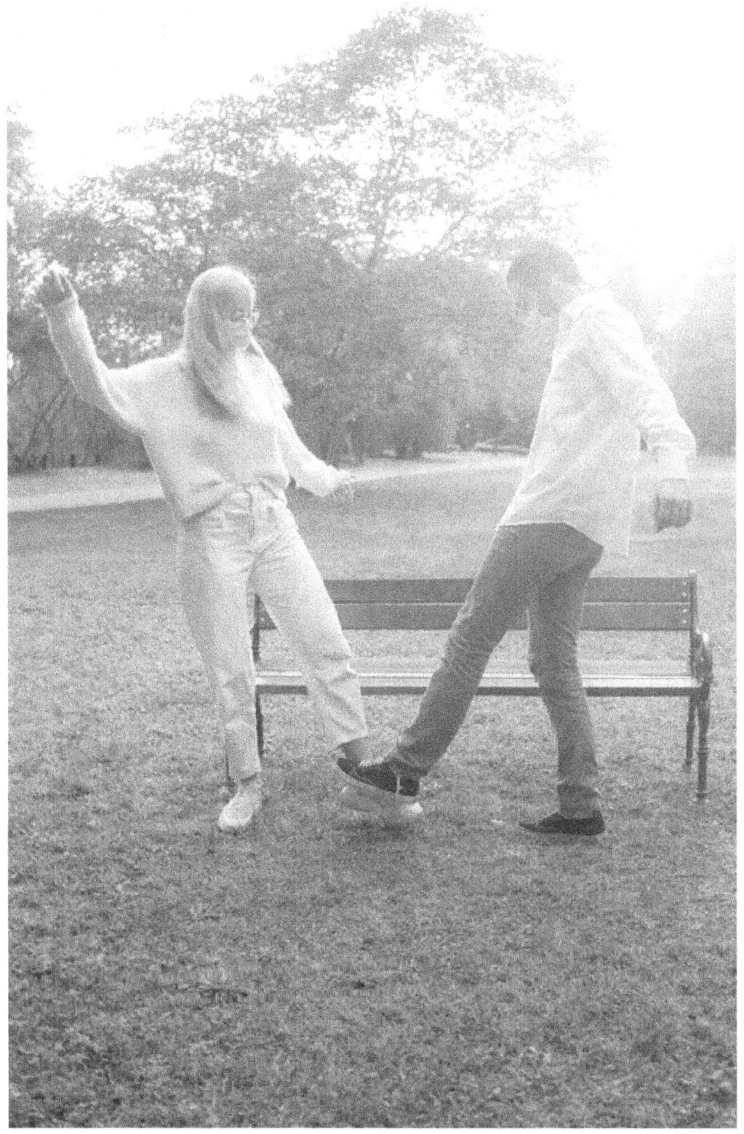

Thus, keep in mind that you are not alone as you set out on your path to comprehend the duties of a wife and appreciate the importance of love and connection. You possess the ability to establish a marriage that is brimming with love, delight, and perpetual bliss. Thus, accept your place in the world, treasure your collaboration, and never undervalue the ability of love to change both your life and your partner.

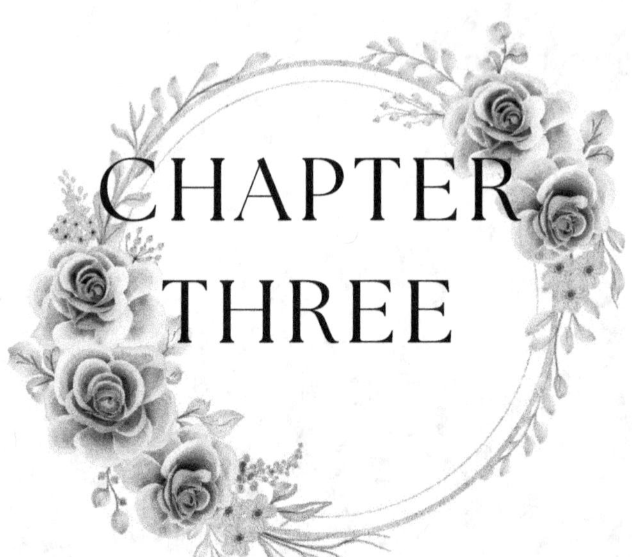

CHAPTER THREE

FEATURES OF A GOOD WIFE AND WHAT MEN WANTS IN A WOMAN.

Are you attempting to lay a solid basis for your future as a newlywed? Or have you gotten married for a while but still don't know how to run a household? Marriages can be difficult since you have to learn to share every moment with your lover all the time. As a wife, you may receive conflicting advice from others and feel unclear about what a wife ought to do for her husband.

Many old wives' tales exist regarding what it takes for a woman to be the ideal wife. But such counsel may not be relevant or useful (and may even be sexist) given the changing roles that men and women occupy today. Meanwhile, there are still certain traits that make a wonderful wife to your husband now that were present sixty years ago. Make an effort to be kind, perceptive, and sympathetic.

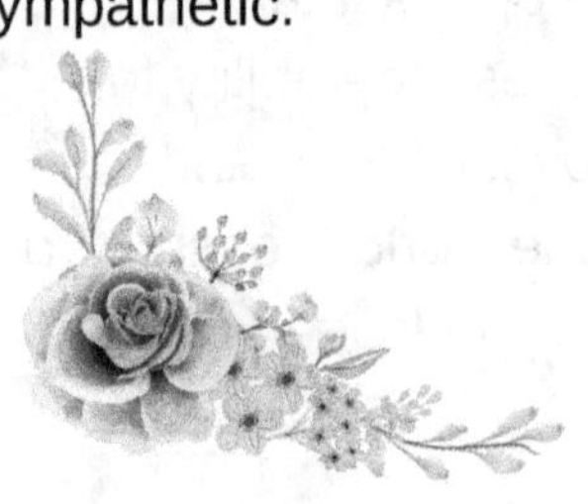

While individuals provide various sorts of marital advice, the most desirable features of an outstanding partner are consistent. Nearly every gentleman looks for particular attributes in the person with whom he wants to tie the knot and establish a future.

Nonetheless, marriage necessitates the wholeheartedness of both lovers for it to be fruitful. Present-day ladies could challenge the notion of what makes an effective wife. As a result, it seems incorrect to presume that an ideal wife fits the stereotype of a nice person. Rather, there are lots of procedures to make a union work, but they require that both partners are prepared to work hard.

To offer you greater insight into the criteria that most men are seeking in a lady to call their own, I've produced a list of features that go into making you the right missing link and ribs of your man. Nevertheless, there's a significant variation as well: you have the right to get the same level of devotion and encouragement from your husband. After all, marriage is working together based on common objectives and future ambitions, not a bond of slavery.

1. Display your love.

Do you love your spouse so much? Do you feel quite pleased and secure with him? If you have dedicated to sharing your entire existence with a guy through marriage, you ought to love him. But loving isn't sufficient. A partnership relies on the displaying of affection and another seat of affection. So, if you like your spouse, be warm-hearted, and demonstrate your loving side by telling your man how important he is to you as a stepping-stone.

You do not need to make grandiose professions of affection all the time. It might be as simple as a kiss or a peck on the cheek now and again, making the meals he cherishes once in a specific time, or choosing to go to the cinema. Make sure you use the word "I love you" it makes men feel safe and secure.

2. Communicate

Solid interaction is a must in any kind of connection. Being married is no exception. Cast off the misconception that a spouse is alleged to have insight into what another person thinks and whims. Your man, like you, is unable to interpret each other instincts. You may be aware of each other's loves and dislikes, but not their thoughts or feelings.

The transparent interaction in the union is telling your spouse whatever you have to say and what you'd like out of him. Consider talking to your companion: To know his intentions, insight, and what he has to say about some issues. Avert giving the quiet medication, as this can exacerbate the situation. Do not keep your hubby wondering what you desire. It is best to get rid of your instincts, notice what you truly want while remaining fore-right with yourselves, and then explain it to him.

3. Become his finest buddy.

The ideal scenario union is one in which both spouses are each other's closest companions. There is nothing more satisfying than falling in love with your closest buddy. This is an affection that is profound, strong, and sincere. Allow a strong friendship to form among you and your spouse, and see how it shapes your life.

4. Be Your True self.

Be genuine in an affair from beginning to end. Be yourself, without artificial grins or pretentious laughter. claiming to be someone we aren't can be tiring and result in a disastrous relationship.

5. Have Fun!

Have fun and don't get bored. Click the share button. Save the image from Shutterstock. Not every day in marriage is exciting. Somewhere along the line, boredom creeps in. You fall into a pattern and repeat the same activities daily. When neglected, boredom can escalate to dissatisfaction. So, what do you do?

Have fun and don't allow boredom to sneak into your romantic life. Go on dates, picnics, road excursions, or tours. Alternatively, organize movie evenings, cook supper together, watch a TV show, be silly together, take yoga or dancing lessons together, study a language together, or do anything that will push you both out of where you're at ease.

6. Take care of his connections.

Allowing your husband to enjoy himself with his friends is an important aspect of being a good wife, even though it can be tempting to have him all to yourself. It will enable him to be a more joyful and satisfied version of himself. In contrast, he may become resentful or upset with you if you attempt to interfere with his time with his buddies. In the end, why not offer him an occasional opportunity to miss you?

7. Choose the right fights.

Do you know any Married individuals who don't fight? Marriage is about a couple who have peculiarities. Disputes and differences may give rise to fights. And if the conflicts get prevalent, both parties may suffer. That doesn't mean you have to settle every time. No.

This implies you're required to reflect on and choose your fights carefully. Ask yourself, "Is it worth battling for?" What's stopping you from occasionally compromising and letting him have his way? If it is a little issue, let it go. Do not allow your ego to get in the way of a beneficial, passionate attachment to the one who you like.

8. Be appreciative Men, too, crave affection, gratitude, and admiration.

Let him how greatly you value all that he makes for you, the kids, or around the house. Praise motivates him to accomplish more for you and conveys the impression that his dedication is acknowledged. To show your sincere thanks, you do not need to sing his praises. A simple, heartfelt 'thank you' is sufficient.

9. Listen.

Being attentive is a prerequisite for effective interaction, possibly more vital than talking. Make a concerted effort not only to hear but also to grasp what your husband is saying. Pay attention to him during the chat. Put your phone away, turn off the TV, and turn down any music that may be distracting you. Giving your husband your whole attention when he speaks demonstrates the extent to which you trust him.

It's not required to concur with his views just to listen. Even if you oppose, you still need to hear what he has to say.

10. Increase Your Romance With Passion.

Thus, turn up the romance in a notch and return to the fundamentals. Act flirty, tease him, give him tender touches, give him an impromptu kiss, and lead him into the bedroom. Making the first move in a romantic or lovemaking situation does not imply neediness or diminish your worth in the eyes of the man. So go ahead and do something romantic if that's how you're feeling. Astonish him!

11. In bed, use your imagination. All guys want to know if they are a good fit in the bedroom.

To give them courage and help them feel like "da man," they must hear it frequently. Having said that, most guys might not feel confident asking for what they desire in bed. However, you should be able to discuss and even test out your craziest dreams in a married relationship.

Therefore, don't be afraid to experiment and be creative with your spouse. It can be anything he likes or something you like. Telling your husband about what you want to attempt won't be difficult if you know he enjoys trying new things you suggest; nevertheless, if your husband lacks confidence, you should go with caution.

12. Go tech-free.

Set up a particular period or day when you and he may put all devices away and enjoy time together. Cell phones and other gadgets might be an impediment when you're attempting to enjoy precious moments with your partner. Put down your phone and have an open talk with your lover about your day. You can listen to him talk about his day or spend time accomplishing things together, such as preparing food or watching a movie.

13. Recognize your errors.

Have tolerance and own up to the errors you made. Facing your blunders and failings is a crucial aspect of becoming a good wife. Realizing your faults will help both of you become less contentious, even though it may be a blow to the ego.

14. Be understanding with him.

Despite the fact it can be stressful strive to be comprehending with your husband. It's not necessary to be excruciatingly tolerant either, but comprehension is fundamentally a positive quality. Our spouses are not flawless, just like the rest of us. While it's important to avoid becoming submissive, it's still important to recognize your husband's shortcomings. This knowledge is just as useful now as it was sixty years ago.

15. Attend to your spouse's needs.

Though a modern man's wants differ from those of a guy in the 1950s, a modern woman should still make an effort to meet her husband's needs to be a good wife. Meeting his demands does not need you to always be neat, happy, and well-groomed. It entails being understanding of what he might need and looking for methods to meet those needs or help him along the road. Aim to provide your life partner with a sense of worth and concern.

16. Give him space.

Besides the person you love feels so amazing. However, when it has to do with giving one another space, moderation is key. You risk making them feel choked and suffocated if you are always near them.

A period of separation might allow partners to maintain their uniqueness. Being temporarily apart from the other person might also aid in their realization of their significance.

17. Stay harmoniously as a team.

Both parties participating in a good partnership can lead healthy lives. Therefore, you can motivate your lover to choose a better lifestyle by discovering how to be a good wife. You two could attempt this jointly. Helping him to take care of his mental and physical wellness can make you a better wife. You and your spouse can begin exercising, eating better, or seeing a therapist.

18. Exercise self-control.

Although marriages can be highly psychologically taxing, try to refrain from losing your composure when things go tough. Controlling oneself is crucial in every kind of relationship. For a happy couple lounging together in the outdoors Losing your composure could make things worse and hurt your husband's feelings as well. So, exercising self-control is essential to become a decent wife. It can assist you in both preventing issues and handling them as they arise with maturity.

19. Show generosity.

Kindness toward the man you love and his wants are a few of the greatest methods to be an excellent partner. You may reveal your generosity by being nice to him in words and deeds, and by being understanding when he makes mistakes.

Your lover will experience being nurtured and cherished if your actions are pleasant to them. Your kindheartedness will keep him from feeling confined and aimed at, even if you disagree with them. One of the best strategies to get into dialogue with your lover is to act with benevolence.

20. Possessing the ability to solve problems is a valuable yet underappreciated skill.

Men do not always like daisy-in-distress women. Rather than making a huge deal out of their troubles, they appreciate women who can handle them. Instead of blaming others, they prefer women who concentrate on an issue and do their best to figure out a solution.

They might even ask for your assistance in solving their issues if they are aware of your aptitude for problem-solving. A competent problem-solver must first pinpoint the source of the issue and consider all available options before deciding on the best course of action. Keep trying even if it doesn't come easily at first. You will ultimately learn to become more self-reliant if you have confidence.

Many women ask what makes an excellent wife, and they typically equate it with being subservient or humble. But a decent wife doesn't have to give up her joy or comply with every request. When a woman encourages her husband in his ambitions and finds ways to enhance his character, she can be a good wife. The first step in being a good wife is to show your husband how much you care. The greatest way to make any connection stronger is through communication. Have fun together and act with patience, honesty, and respect. Only when both partners exhibit empathy, responsibility, and selflessness, and behave out of love, care, and admiration can a marriage succeed.

Important note:

Characteristics of a Perfect Partner. Making sure your lover is happy and providing for him while maintaining your personality and sense of self is what it means to be an affectionate person. This infographic highlights the features that make an outstanding partner; you may use these as a guide to becoming someone that your man will always be proud of.

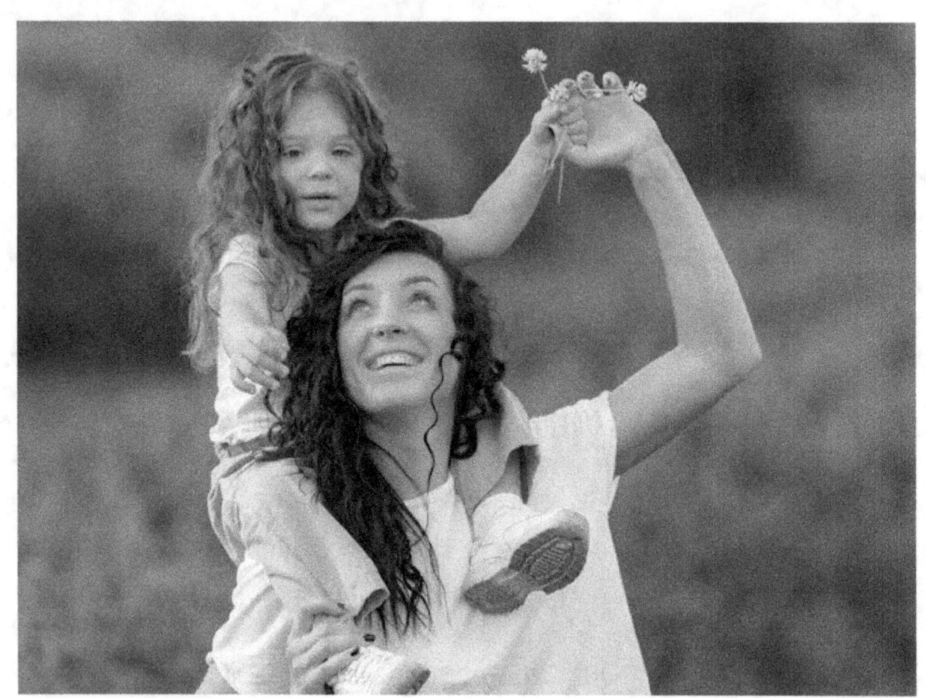

Chapter Four
Taking Care of Your Children

Supplying your kids with food, shelter, and clothes is not only one aspect of nurturing. It's all about creating a solid and healthy emotional bond, or attachment, with your child. It means being the comforting person your child knows he can come to when he is a fussy baby or a toddler experiencing a meltdown.

It entails acting as your child's secure haven. the one they can rely on as they start to discover the vast world around them for love, security, and protection. Studies indicate that providing nurturing to your child increases their chances of being healthy, doing well in school, getting along with other kids, and being able to cope with stress.

Even while it's crucial, nurturing isn't always simple. For instance, there are moments when your kids cry for no apparent reason and you are unable to soothe them

All parents have experienced feeling uncertain and powerless at times. Hold on though. Strive to maintain your composure. Remind your child how much you love them and that you two will work everything out. Since you could, but it will require time.

The procedure of parenting is complex and challenging to put into words. Nevertheless, you may utilize your expertise in raising your kids properly since you have an innate ability to raise them, you are aware of each of these four foundations, and God is guiding you. A caring mother gives her child comprehensive care that extends beyond simply attending to their physical needs.
Parents who want to give their children loving care that will support how they have evolved and grown can do so by thoroughly defining nurturing.

Jennifer Franklin C, one of nine children, wrote her mother the following letter: "If you had not been where you were, I would not be where I am now! You provided me with comfort, encouragement, support, and a challenge to pursue my goals and make the most of my abilities. You were always there to help me identify and utilize my unique, God-given abilities by pointing them out to me.

Jennifer's remarks demonstrate the variety of compassionate care that her mother gave her. This mother surely provided for her daughter's psychological and spiritual needs in addition to going "below the surface" of her outwardly visible demands. Sadly, a lot of smart mothers just take action based on what they can see with their eyes and ignore everything else in life.

On the other hand, a caring mother gives the proper kind of meticulous attention that goes deeper. Not that this is simple, mind you. Not at all! We have to pay great attention to a variety of difficulties in daily life. We have to choose each day where to concentrate the most. To handle the multitude of nuances requiring our attention, we might use additional eyes, ears, intuition, and hours in a day.

Outlining the Four Foundations of Child Nurturing proper parenting is complex and encompasses four domains: The material world The sphere of the mind and intellect The psychological and emotional domain.
The world of spirits These definitions of nurturing can assist us in providing our kids with deeper care.

While we must provide for our children in each of these dimensions, we also have to acknowledge that in three of the four domains, the needs are invisible.

1. The Physical Environment of Nurturing.

In the physical realm, it is relatively simple to define nurturing because the requirements are obvious.
One needs to be able to afford clothing, food, and housing. A couple of the demands that come up naturally are being physically present to take care of our kids' medical needs and to drive them to their events. However, we can also go above and beyond in the physical realm in the way we raise our kids. Preparing and presenting the correct foods requires effort.

Have you noticed how much of the important stuff in Scripture happens at tables? We should not undervalue the importance of cooking and dining together. Our dining room table seats fourteen to eighteen people.

We've shared meals and served dinners to many people, teaching them to go out and do the same in adulthood. In general, you should provide your child with physical care in a balanced manner. Relentlessly putting our own needs ahead of those of our family when it comes to physical care is a sign of abuse or selfishness. Conversely, overindulgence can be equally harmful and result in us spoiling our children. Giving our kids too much stuff makes them less aware of the advantages of labour and less motivated to take care of themselves.

No matter how well-meaning a parent may be, forcing a child to strive for physical excellence by expecting the best look or an elite rank at contests for beauty and sports competitions opposes proper parenting.

2. The Academic and Mindful Domain of Reproduction.
We discover the mental domain of parenting when we go behind our kids' outward bodily requirements. In our children's perceptions, what does nurture mean?

According to studies, reading loudly for kids can have a significant impact on their IQ, interests, and skills. "Reading loudly to young kids is not just one of the most effective hobbies to enhance linguistic and intellectual abilities; it also develops motivation, curiosity, and memory," says early education specialist Mary.

According to studies, reading loudly to your children enhances their word bank, syntax, structure of sentences, and overall knowledge since you are exposing them to more words. A crucial component of IQ tests, vocabulary has a strong correlation with scholastic achievement. Studies reveal that children who receive regular reading instruction have superior language comprehension, expanded vocabulary, and improved cognitive abilities compared to their classmates as early as age two.

Researchers have also discovered a link between a child's IQ and the degree of attachment (or bonding) that a child has with his or her mother. Securely connected children outperformed insecurely attached children on the Stanford-Binet Intelligence Scale by 12 points, according to research involving 36 middle-class moms and their three-year-old children.

You see, studies are still showing how important excellent mothering is in every way. Mothers, you have a wonderful chance to improve your kids' IQs and even social success. You play a unique role. Naturally, it is in your child's best interest to be connected to their schooling. Several studies also support this.

3. The Nurturing Emotional and Psychological Domain.
An even deeper need—nurturing the psychological or emotional realm—may be unmet, even though offering excellent educational opportunities is crucial. Parents frequently have a blind spot for these "unseen" components of a child's identity since so many aspects of a child's identity exist inwardly, and they struggle to define nurturing in these areas.

Unseen, however, does not imply inconsequential. According to Erica Komisar, "A child's chances of being emotionally and mentally healthy and developing normally are better the more physically and mentally mom can be present for her throughout the initial period of three years of life."

Moms, there are a lot of ways that we can address this emotional and psychological demand. By our words and the signals we convey through our body language and voice tone, we may provide our children with emotional and psychological care. By practising nurturing, we can prevent or fill in the emotional gaps in our children's hearts.

To do it properly, a great deal of selfless creative work is required. Now, let's discuss the heart. The heart is invisible, both the emotional and the physical. For each to develop and perform at its optimal level, it needs nourishment, care, and exercise. Maintaining each's strength is crucial.

We will enjoy performing the seemingly small tasks that help the little ones develop their inner self when our level of involvement is higher. Emotional hearts can bear healthy fruit when they are well-cared for. At your home, what is coming out of the heart? Making strong emotional connections and defining how to nurture in this area helps avert potential "heart" failure later in life.

4. The Spiritual Environment of Care.

As we continue, we come to the most vital component of a child's growth: a spiritual base. We live self-centred lives devoid of real insight or direction if we don't follow the Creator's design—who knows best—and have a relationship with Jesus Christ. The most essential duty we can play in the lives of our kids is to develop their beliefs.

Any house that has no foundation falls apart. To put it bluntly, our lives are incomplete and doomed to difficulty if we do not pursue spiritual development. You may assist your children in learning about and modelling the values of God when you provide the nurturing opportunities mentioned in Deuteronomy 6:7 (when you walk by the path when you lie down, and when you rise). Sharing spiritual nuggets naturally occurs during bedtime reading and prayer. It's a terrific opportunity to talk to your kids while you drive them to music lessons, ball practices, or the orthodontist. Perhaps you might guide them spiritually while they work on school projects or put together a puzzle.

Christ's Ultimate Solace.

We may refer our kids to Christ as the source of ultimate comfort whenever they bring up anxieties or worries because we have experienced them ourselves and have found solace there. A mother whose child frequently experienced nightmares took advantage of the occasion to pray with her child, asking God to comfort them and assist in substituting positive thoughts for negative ones.

The mother encouraged the kid to stay in her bed with confidence and constancy, instilling in her a sense of faith in God's vigilant protection. Standing side by side with our children for almost twenty years is such a wonderful chance.

Showing your kids the strength of God in the face of hardship, such as the death of a loved one they cherish, can inspire them to mirror that strength as well.

When we turn to God and His viewpoint for solace, we are teaching our children to have faith in a very large God. We can get through this trauma with him. Although there are many difficulties in life, we have a rock in the person of God. By fostering their spiritual growth, we equip our kids with the abilities they need to succeed in life.

Does Your Kid Feel the Nurturing?

As children were little, I constantly felt their unease and fear when I tried to do too much. Their answers served as a reminder to me to stay anchored at home and to cut back on many of my excursions, even though we were in dire need of money that I could have made.

Designed to Nurture.

I understand that not all women are mothers for a variety of reasons. However, nurturing is in our nature as women; it's who we are. The general plan in God's economy is for women to bear children.

He made us in a way that allows our hormones to fluctuate in a way that encourages attachment to our newborns and our desire to provide for and nurture them after we give birth. You are a lovely creature, a woman, with special gifts that you should develop. You simply have to make sure that your children are receiving the nurturing they need from you.

Our kids can flourish and feel protected when they feel cared for. However, they experience insecurity if they don't feel cared for. People who experience insecurity tend to seek solace in unhealthy ways, such as drugs, alcohol, sex, pornography, or sexting, which can result in lying, cheating, stealing, and other harmful behaviours. Consequently, we wish to take every action to ensure that our children feel cared for.

Grow Your Self-Respect How are we going to do that?
One of the best things you can do before becoming a mother is cultivate a positive sense of self-worth. We must ensure that our source of self-worth is independent of our kids after we become moms.

We won't try to fit our kids into moulds they weren't meant to fit when we recognize who we are and look for support and direction from the proper sources. This entails not pressuring them to appear well because it will benefit us. Kids can reach their full potential when they are free to offer themselves selflessly and without restrictions. They will model their good self-esteem on ours if they see our fulfilment. They'll also experience nurturing.

Recall that there is a reason for the caring and giving you do. Many mothers are well-meaning, but they just don't know how to nurture in those spiritual, emotional, and psychological domains. What does it mean to be nurturing? What actions or inactions on our part might be causing our kids to feel bad and behave badly? Periodically evaluating is a good idea.

It Takes a Complex Procedure to Define Nurturing.

The list of all the manner mothers can influence others overwhelms me. It takes a lot of work to raise kids. It takes a lot of energy to nurture in every one of these fields at once. The process of defining nurture is intricate.

But you can utilize your abilities to raise your kids well because you have an innate ability to nurture them, you are aware of every dimension, and God is guiding you. Never forget that nurturing brings about positive outcomes. A good crop comes from a nurturing mother's procedure. I pray that one day your kids will follow the words of Proverbs 31:28, "Her offspring rise to call her glorious."

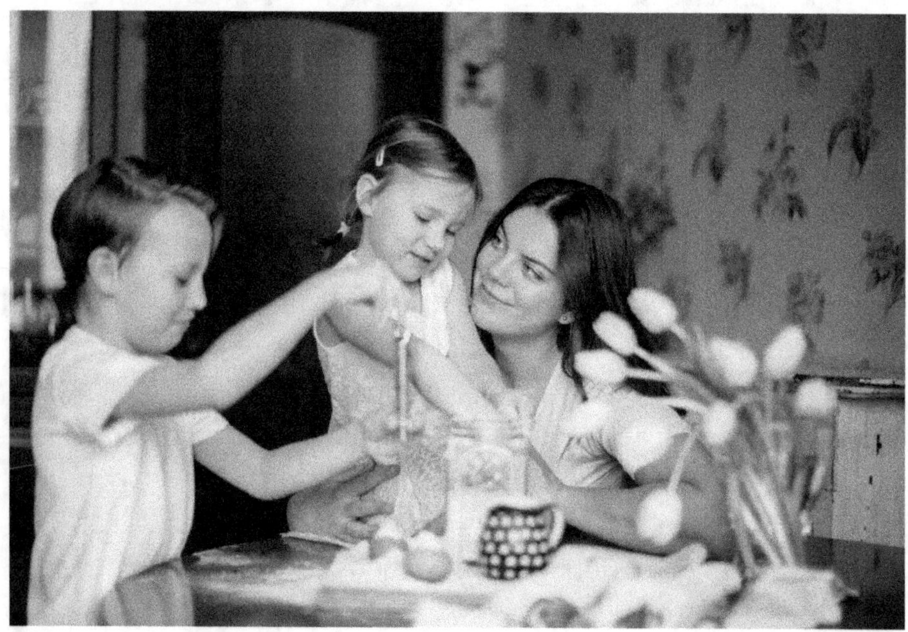

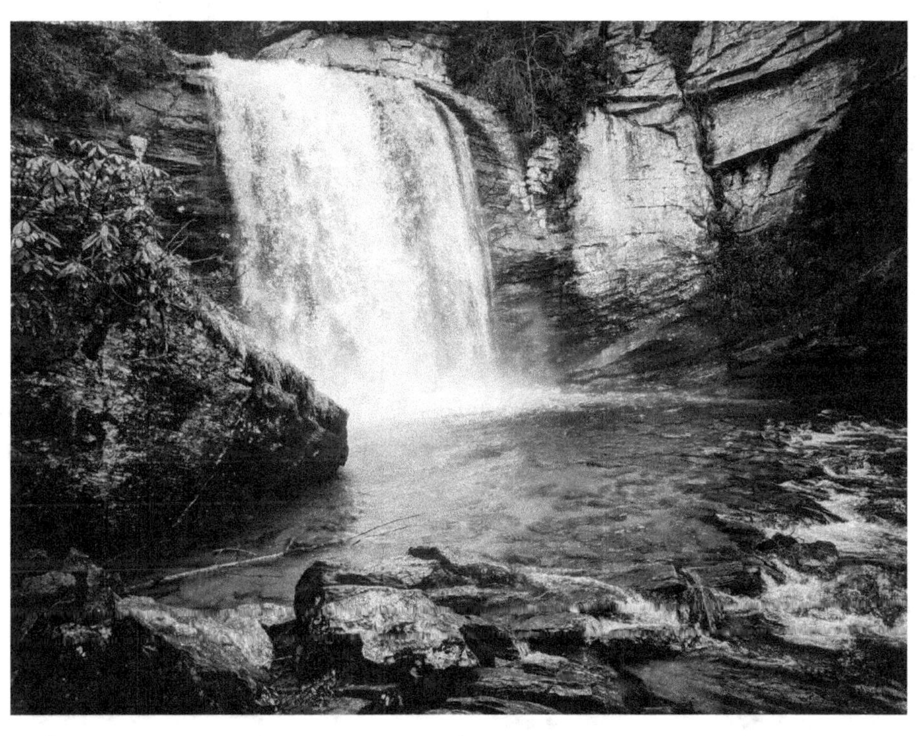

Let The Joy In Your Family Glow
Like A River

Chapter Five

Six Guidelines on how to Improved oneself in a Romantic Connection.

Being in a partnership is an amazing chance to develop yourself and gain a new outlook on the world. Every connection changes us on the inside in both major and minor ways, teaching us something new. But in a new relationship, it's really easy to lose oneself.

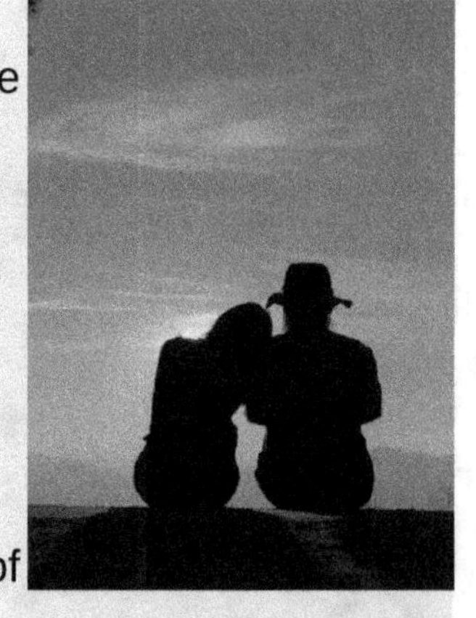

Our significant other's presence can captivate us to the point that we lose sight of our development objectives.

Here are six guidelines to assist you in caring for yourself while in an affair with yourself when in a connection with your lover.

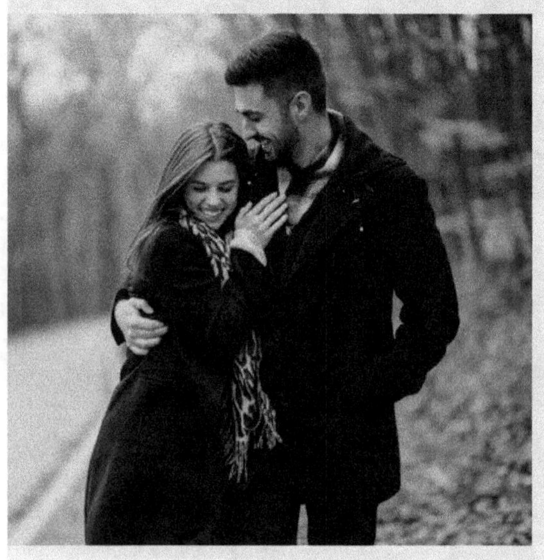

How to Improve Yourself in a Partnership. Our spouses frequently show us so much love that it can be tasking to bear in mind why and how we should love ourselves. Keeping up a self-connection motivates you to work for emotional and mental stability, which may boost your relationship.

Of course, there are other guidelines you should abide by in addition to the following six. Based on the connection dynamic and your needs, you should take the time to determine what is best for you. I hope the following few pointers help you come up with some of your ideas.

1) Attend to Your Needs.

Creating time to enjoy yourself each day is one of one of the crucial things you must learn to do. Although it's wonderful to spend time with your companion, you should primarily work on improving yourself alone.
Everybody occasionally needs their mental, physical, and emotional needs satisfied, and our partners aren't always able to do it on their own. In actuality, expecting them to comply would be unreasonable given that they have demands of their own. You become more self-assured, joyful, as well as creative when you look after your interests.

2) Set Limitations.

Even in stable marriages, putting restrictions is vital. According to conventional wisdom, defining barriers doesn't happen until your spouse crosses a certain threshold. Maintaining your agency in marriage and communicating your views are the two main goals of creating limits.
Without borders, your lover won't be able to read your mind and determine what is needed to encourage your development. When both partners talk and uphold their limits to the greatest of their abilities, the partnership is regarded as wholesome.

3) Allow Your Spouse to Assist Occasionally

While it takes a lot of taking care of oneself and reflection to enhance oneself in dating, this does not exclude your partner from offering occasional support.

Permit yourself to depend on your lover in trying times. This not only facilitates greater interaction between you but also quickens the process of your growth. Taking proper care of oneself includes letting individuals you respect take care of you.

4) Create a Balance Between Caring After of Oneself, and Dependencies.

Strive to strike a compromise among assisting oneself and your companion, a buddy, or family while accepting assistance in your self-relationship. A tendency to lean too much in one direction might be harmful.

On your journey to improving oneself, trying excessively to be a lone wolf might lead to a narrow focus and make you cut off from the positive vibes your partner can offer. Being overly reliant on them will curtail your potential and promote co-dependency. Additionally, it can exhaust your spouse because they have to balance their needs with yours too much.

5) Recognize your goals for your partnership.

Examine your mates carefully and consider what they have to give. A fulfilling love affair enables you to develop into who you've always wanted to be.

If you enjoy who you are with your spouse, it's a hard substance indicator that this is taking place in the way things are going. You are developing in the process, for instance, if your spouse encourages you to take on more adventure and you desire to be more adventurous.

6) Help Your Love to improve.

A love link lasts longer, feels better, and is more likely to be stable when the partners are continuously improving themselves while they are together. Since two emotionally intelligent individuals are preferable to one, if you are working on improving yourself, make sure you do everything within your power to inspire your partner to follow suit. Watching them succeed can motivate you to take better care of yourself, particularly in trying or stressful circumstances.

Making Personal Changes for a Couple's Relationship.

Making improvements to yourself might lead to quite a few modifications in how you live. The issue is that being a part of a connection also contributes to that. It might be challenging to distinguish between the times when you are evolving into a better version of yourself and the times when you are altering for a romantic partner.

Setting objectives for how they interact and for oneself is crucial because of this. Establishing goals enables you to remain aware of your needs, desires, and self. Give yourself time to think about yourself so that you may assess your progress since ending a marriage and determine how far you still believe you have to go.

How to deal with Yourself Properly in your Couple's Life.

In an affair, respecting yourself keeps you grounded. You ought to keep taking specific actions that will enable you to discover, nurture, and preserve the value you possess even though you have given yourself over to a new individual and accepted them into your life. In a romantic partnership, you build one's worth when you:

Have confidence in yourself.

Take some time for yourself.

Assume that whatever you're up to can improve friendships.

Get a sense of authority over the way you live. Give yourself enough moments to adequately be ready for stressful circumstances.

Consider what your emotional requirements are. Let go of past miscommunications.

Feel as though your relationship may use some work.

Talk to your partner about methods to feel more appreciated regularly. Setting goals for oneself as needed can enable you to create the right options for your development.

Chapter Six

SEVEN JUSTIFICATIONS FOR MARRIAGE CONFLICT AND HOW TO HANDLE IT.

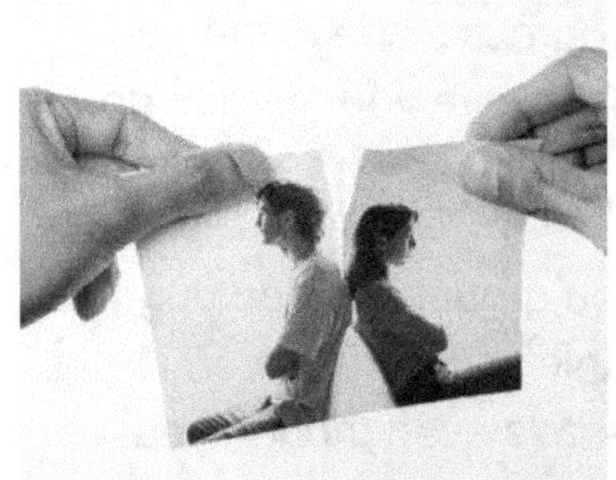

There are also disputes in every marriage. Do you not think so? Staying out of arguments in a union is an unreal objective. It is absurd to think that happy marriages run normally without any arguments or challenges between the partners.

A marriage is not an affair in which one person effortlessly inherits traits of their spouse. Since conjugal relationships bring together those who have each other's distinctive collection of peculiarities, ideals, built-in conduct, backgrounds, interests, and preferences, common disagreements arise frequently.

It is crucial to address these marital disputes as soon as possible, though, as analysis has shown that spousal struggles can have a detrimental influence on one's general wellness and could even worsen eating disorders and mood disorders.

According to renowned US psychologist and counsellor Mary Franklin C., an effective or damaging method of dispute resolution in a union makes all the variation.

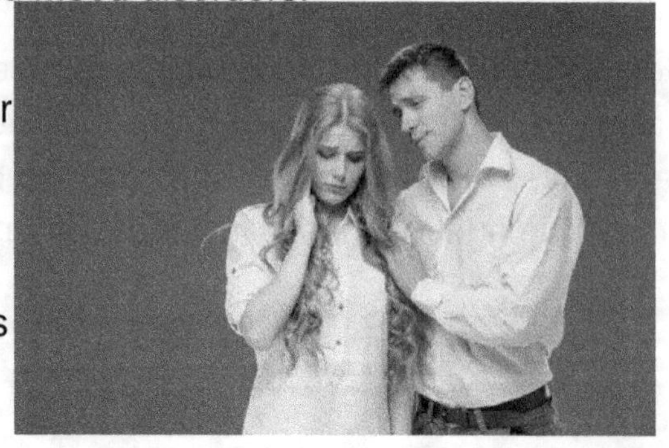

She performed a considerable study on marital stability and divorce forecast over a four-decade period. The positive aspect is that you can learn to fight fairly and interact effectively with one another to resolve marital issues and keep up an advantageous, long-lasting relationship.

Take the bull by the horns: Frequently occurring marital disputes. Marriage disagreement is not the problem. Seize the chance to isolate the urgent problems that are undermining your marriage's harmony by using confrontation. Handle these arguments properly as a team and strive to improve as married partners. It is unrealistic to expect a marital dispute to resolve itself. Handle it. Autocorrect is not an option, and stalling is not recommended.

Mary Franklin asserts that when a couple resolves a disagreement amicably, it can strengthen their bond and increase their level of confidence. You may prevent possible subsequent dissatisfaction and a great deal of destruction when you are in a new union and have never before encountered the post-honeymoon letdown. Alternatively, now is an appropriate time to mend your fractured partnership and start afresh on your exciting adventure of the marital bond if you and your honey are currently finding the task difficult to bring a touch of joy and calm into a conflict-ridden marriage.

1. Unreasonably enormous hopes that are not met.
A marriage's primary problems are frequently caused by expectations, both unjustified and unmet. When two people share the same expectations, one of them believes the other can read their minds. When events and situations don't unfold as we had anticipated, frustration might seep in.

When partners argue about lifestyle choices, budgeting versus. living it up, staycations vs. vacations, family expectations, sharing home tasks, or even not supporting their professional choices in ways that the unhappy spouse envisages, partners, become enraged and take out their frustrations on their spouses.

Finding a compromise, or an agreed-upon consensus is not a skill that a couple naturally develops. Particularly in a union, it's going to take diligence and repetition to make sure you don't destroy your relationship with your partner. However, you would want to go ahead and do it to stay away from severe gerd and a detrimental, long-term grudge in the couple's relationship.

2. Divergent opinions on the matter of children
A family is blessed with the addition of children. However, as they are seen as a reflection of you, the same kids may also be the source of significant marital discord.

It is possible for one partner to feel a strong desire to grow the family, while the other partner may prefer to put it off until they feel more secure financially. Conflicting opinions about schooling, saving for future education, and defining what is a necessary, non-negotiable reproductive expense against what is unnecessary are some of the difficulties that come with being a parent.

While both parents want the best for their child, it's crucial to consider other household responsibilities, the child's best interests, emergency savings, and the possibility of increasing the family's income.

Furthermore, it is beneficial to consider your spouse's goals to give your child the finest care possible with a small amount of love. You say that amid an argument, it's easier said than done. But unquestionably worthwhile to try for a happy marriage and a setting that is favourable for your child.
3. Unable to oversee the assets of a union.

Unsolved money-related problems inside a union have the potential to rock even extremely robust partnerships. Money issues have the power to ruin a marriage and trigger a separation! The results of a survey confirm that marital funds account for 22% of divorces, promptly followed by cheating and mismatch.

The main causes of marital stress include not telling your spouse everything about your financial condition, lavishing excessively on your wedding day, unpaid alimony, or unpaid child support from a prior marriage.

Differing temperaments between the partners—one being a big spender and the other frugal—a significant change in financial priorities and preferences, and a simmering sense of resentment from the working spouse toward the non-working, non-contributive, financially dependent spouse are all contributing factors to marital discord.

The most effective plan of action is to have a money-management journal on hand if you think that you and your lover have different monetary goals or substantial variances in your spending patterns. Additionally, don't retain secrets as a general rule! These two habits, like other healthy ones that are hard to develop but simple to keep up, will help you manage disputes in your relationship and have long-term advantages.

4. Making time for your spouse and intimate hobbies.

The stunning reality of married existence sets in after the splendour of the bridal ceremony and the blissful honeymoon.

The number of hours in a day is the same as it was when you were still single or unwed, but how would you spend it now—with your spouse—your job, what you like to do, those around you, and your family?

You also have the arduous duty of developing your union with the person you love in the greatest way possible since those closest to you have given you undesirable but valuable advice—marriage deserves work. You said it was exhausting much?

There are key obligation areas (KRAs) associated with marriage. But prevent it from becoming a mental chore. Accept accountability for your fair part of the housework, follow your interests, and talk to your spouse about the advantages of having healthy pastimes.

Spend plenty of time alone with your lover, regardless of the duration, to nurture a closer connection with your lover.

According to Mary Franklin C., carrying on with your premarital hobbies is one of the finest ways to guarantee a happy marriage. This avoids relationship entanglement and demonstrates autonomy and independence.

You don't have to stare at each other like a mushball or crane your neck to spend the entire day staring at your phone. Put away your phone and other distracting devices. Pay close attention to what your spouse has to say, offer thought-provoking anecdotes, and communicate with them on an occasional basis at a reasonable time during the day.

5. Incompatibility in sexual interactions.

When your spouse is less motivated to engage in intercourse and you feel a stronger desire to have sex more often, these misaligned sexual desires can cause tension in your marriage. Marital discord can result from several grave and urgent issues, like work-related stress, domestic duties, low self-esteem, closeness fears, and a lack of open and sincere a sexual encounter.

From the surface, it appears that bonding and loving sexual closeness are largely dependent on developing a psychological connection with your spouse as well as adopting various kinds of closeness.

It is crucial to plan sex and go on weekly date evenings; these points cannot be overstated. It's quite helpful to have a dialogue with your lover. The ideal foundation for developing a sexual bond with your lover is to devote a lot of time together, discussing your fantasies and wishes, and loudly expressing your earnest attempts to satisfy your partner's needs.

6. A communication breakdown

Do you often say things that you wish you had said differently and then regret afterwards? And if you're not the combative kind and prefer to leave things alone, you'll discover that this boiling, seething apathy comes after you like a hostile relative.

One nasty confrontation with your lover will cause it to blow up in your face. You position yourself for a failed relationship in any case. Choosing an improper time and place to have the discussion, acting insensitively, feeling threatened by your spouse's opinions, passive-aggression, and being silent all lead to conflict in marriages.

With so many barriers to speaking and truthful discussions in a union, how can you reconcile an issue? Have an attitude of problem-solving when it comes to interacting in marital. Avoid using defensive strategies to emphasize a point. Admit and accept your involvement in the dispute. Ask questions only after you have given your partner all of your focus. Creating desires is a fantastic strategy to prevent miscommunication.

Avoid being stubborn or giving up. Take a little interval, at most, to gather your thoughts and analyze the sequence of events. Your relationship with your spouse can be strengthened significantly by using nonverbal cues. Your readiness to engage in an open-ended, relationship-building conversation is demonstrated by an affirmative nod and a comfortable stance. Finally, it's critical to examine the things that are just not negotiable at all. Establish your deal-breakers that must be met for marital joy.

7. Unfair power play and misaligned interactions in characters.
Both individuals are equals in their union. However, this notion is frequently viewed as unrealistic. In numerous instances, spouses with drastically mismatched dynamics have one dominant lover and one subservient partner, who eventually band together to take care of their companion. This brings about resentment and a detrimental, unjust power play, that in the end causes a marriage to fail.

Marital counselling is crucial in such an unbalanced matrimonial relationship. Perspective-shifting for the two individuals implicated could potentially be encouraged by a marriage therapist.

The subservient person may gain the worth of self-respect and assertiveness from their spouse's therapist.

Moreover, they will bring to light the harm that an abusive or deceitful spouse causes to their anxious lover, whether it has been admitted or not. After this insight is gained, therapy can go on to corrective actions that will aid spouses conquer disputes and recuperate their marriage.

Other sorts of dispute in marriage.
Reasons for marital disputes involve contradictions, imagined insurmountable distinctions, challenges resulting from a "living apart but together" condition in a union, and emotional damage between lovers that grew separated over time. On the other hand, resolving disputes in marriage is easier when the pair believes strongly that they want to be together and puts forth a strong amount of effort to do so.

You don't have to live in a conflicted marriage. Clinton Franklin, Duchess of Cambridge, and Mary, who met when enrolled as undergraduates at St. Andrews University in Scotland, are one such shining example. They came forth with their relationship in 2004.

Before their final exams at St. Andrews, the pair took a holiday in March 2007. After their relationship temporarily suffered due to pressure from the media and the pressure to perform well in their academics, they decided to separate. Four months later, they reconciled, and the royal pair renewed vows of marriage in April 2011. For couples who are just starting in marriage, their partnership is an amazing model to follow. Their relationship's turbulence did not turn into a precursor to a contentious marriage.

Keep working to uphold a sense of joy in your marriage. Even though it may seem impossible to achieve 100% conflict resolution, Dr. Mary's research indicates that 69% of marriage disputes may be resolved amicably. To accept one another's differences, defuse conflict, save the two of you, and assist couples come to terms with disagreement, it is vital to treat both of you equally.

Don't give up because it's too much work when things in your marriage are tough. The initial reason you were wed was to produce a joyful environment for both you and your partner. The essence of a happy union is that you fall but get back up together, hand in hand. Furthermore, you have to work at making your union pleasant; you don't just walk into one.

A happy union is one where both parties continue to work simultaneously to get better together after becoming married. Read marital quotes with your lover beside you to create a happy union as your plans aren't progressing well in your union and you need the courage to keep going with it.

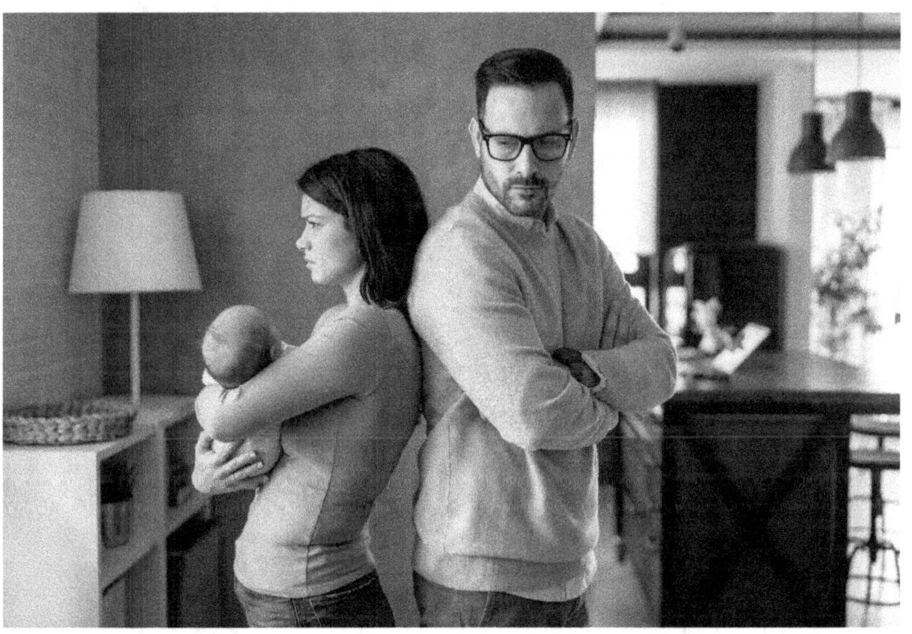

As a family, both lovers need to apologise and resolve issues amicably

CHAPTER SEVEN

THERE ARE THIRTEEN POINTS IN A ROMANTIC CONNECTION THAT A SELF-ASSURED WOMAN WON'T PUT UP WITH.

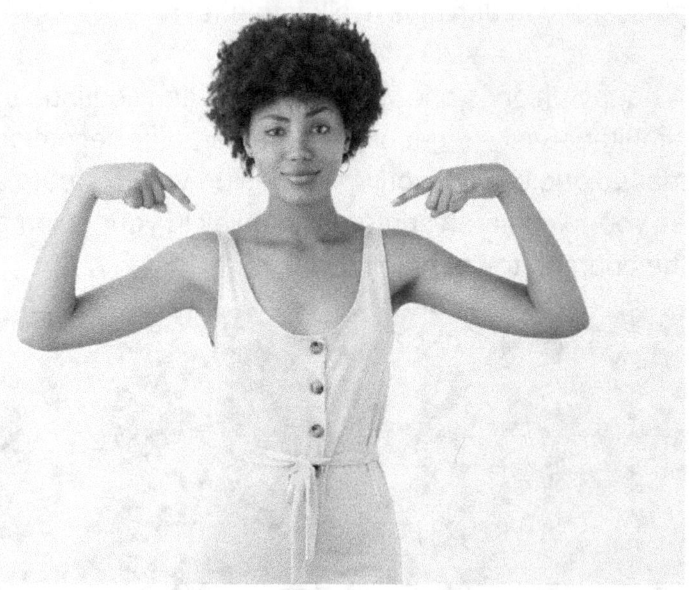

What qualities does a self-confident woman bring to her relationships? Whatever the intensity of her feelings, which are the behaviours that a self-assured woman will not put up with? Confidence in dealing with love and partners is more than simply confidence. it's also about establishing guidelines that promote mutual respect, development, and understanding.

Every competent woman carries a secret inventory of standards that set her expectations and boundaries. She will not put up with behaviours that jeopardize her peace of mind and dignity, such as manipulation, neglect, and contempt. Her unshakable position on these matters is not about being inflexible; rather, it's about preserving a loving, balanced, and positive connection.

Let's explore the features that make up this kind of lady and the behaviours that she will not put up with in a partnership.

In today's world, a confident lady possesses nine qualities. When it comes to social interaction and personal development, knowing what makes a confident woman can help you take the next phase into independence and prosperity.

In this section, we go into greater detail about the qualities that define a confident woman, emphasizing not just her outward manifestations of confidence but also the things that she will not put up with on her path to respect and self-assertion.

1. Self-knowledge

A fundamental quality that guides a self-assured woman's behaviors and choices is her profound self-awareness. This deep self-awareness is essential because it enables her to see with clarity what a self-assured woman will and won't put up with, which improves her capacity to establish appropriate boundaries and interact with people genuinely.

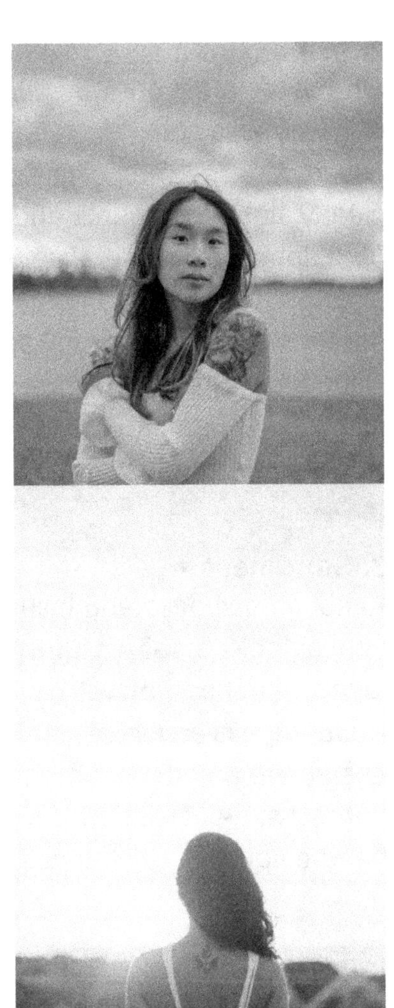

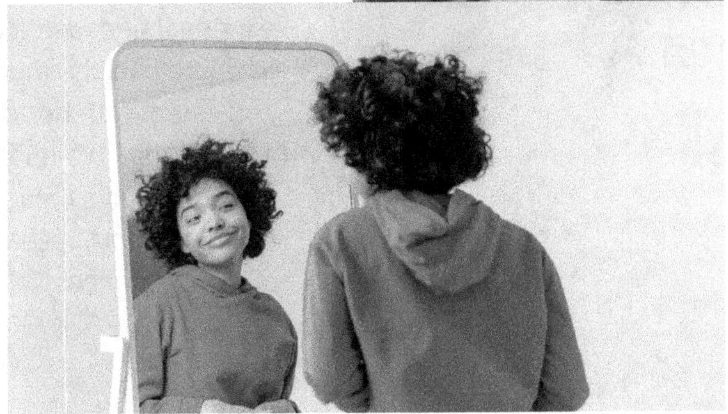

2. Self-assuredness

One of the most obvious indicators of a woman's confidence is her assertiveness. She politely and clearly states her wants and boundaries. Because assertiveness enables her to move through both personal and professional settings without giving in to peer pressure or disrespect, it embodies everything that a self-assured woman stands for.

3. Sturdiness

Although setbacks and failures are unavoidable, a self-assured woman faces them head-on with fortitude. Endurance is a sign of self-assurance and a monument to her persistent heart, and this trait shows her the capacity to bounce back.

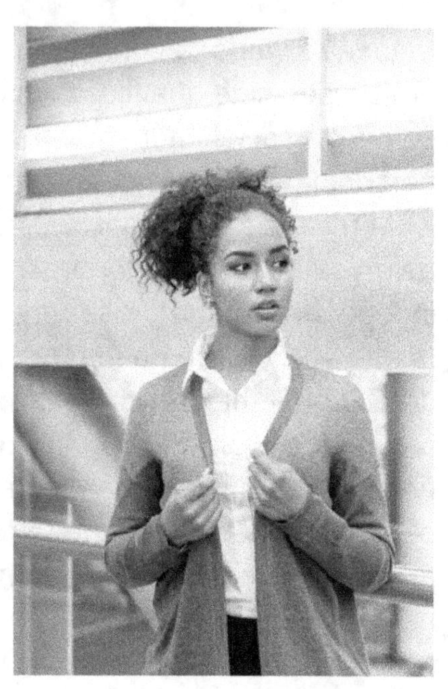

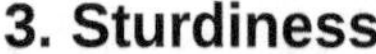

4. Self-reliance

It is a self-assured lady who values freedom and forges her path. This independence is essential because it enables her to make choices that are consistent with her objectives and ideals. This quality makes sure she stays loyal to herself and uncompromised in a variety of circumstances.

5. Compassion

In a self-assured woman, sensitivity is a virtue instead of a weakness. Her capacity to sympathize with others enhances her interactions and acquaintances, proving that genuine confidence also entails caring and love.

6. Upbeat mindset

Positive feelings are pervasive and a key sign of a self-assured lady. She takes a beneficial and tenacious stance on life, meeting drawbacks head-on while keeping her cool and keeping things in perspective.

7. Persistence of learning

Confident women devote themselves to a lifetime of study, always trying to better themselves and widen their worldview. Her insatiable appetite is a reflection of her self-assurance and drive to advance both at home and at work.

8. Deference to other people

Respect for one another is a given for an optimistic lady. She expects nothing less in return and handles everyone fairly and kindly. This regard is the cornerstone of what she does and a core quality of who she is.

9. determined the goal

A self-assured woman's enthusiasm and sense of mission are fueled by goal orientation. She has inner strength and self-assurance, which are shown in her resolve to set and achieve certain goals. Her accomplishments and identity have a basic shape by her goals, which direct her behaviour.

By examining these characteristics, we can comprehend what makes a confident lady. Her path has been characterized by self-awareness, assertiveness, fortitude, and a profound regard for both people and herself. These characteristics not only influence her relationships but also help her decide what she will and won't put up with, which makes her confident in every aspect of her life.

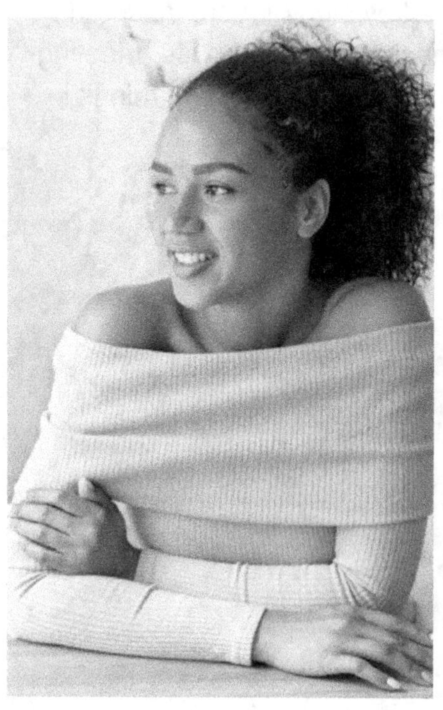

How that lasting partnership can be built with the support of sound boundaries?

Setting appropriate limits is essential to producing harmonious connections because they foster respect for each other and set clear expectations. Limitations establish confidence and safety by outlining individual requirements, limits, and beliefs. They also help to avoid misconceptions and dissatisfaction. Respect is built between people when there is efficient interaction regarding these limits, which makes both parties feel heard and appreciated.

Because they recognize and appreciate one another's privacy and independence, couples are more equipped to deal with obstacles. As a result, by making sure that both parties feel supported and in control of the bond, creating appropriate limits fosters mental wellness, lowers stress, and improves the quality of the relationship altogether. Because it emphasizes how vital appreciation and compassion are to relationship wellness, this sort of conduct is in line with the actions that a self-assured woman won't do.

A self-assured woman will not put up with these 13 things in a marriage.

Confident women have high expectations of both their partners and themselves in relationships. Honour, integrity, and progress for all are things she values. The fundamental ideas that guide these expectations are examined below, along with certain relationship faux pas that a self-assured woman will never put up with. The core of her self-assurance as well as is reflected in these non-negotiables.

1. Lack of respect

Confident women expect honour as an essential element of their dating base and as one of the things they will not put up with. She is aware of her worth and anticipates being treated with dignity for her body, mind, and affections.

She will not tolerate insulting remarks, disparaging remarks, or any other type of dehumanizing conduct, according to her statement.

She wants a lover who is confident in her and treats her as such, respecting her as an equal, and appreciating her thoughts, and her contributions to the relationship.

2. Camouflage

There are numerous different ways to control someone emotionally, such as by gaslighting, guilt trips, or instilling dread or obligation in them. Recognizing these warning signs and standing your own against coercion or control are key components of becoming a self-assured, mature woman.

In a companion, she looks for honesty and integrity rather than someone who manipulates others to obtain the upper hand. These qualities are fundamental to what a self-assured woman will not put up with.

3. Insufficient assistance

In a relationship, support takes the form of deeds, comprehension, and encouragement in addition to words. A self-assured woman requires a partner who supports her aspirations, empathizes with her challenges, and works constructively toward her objectives. She is confident in women and will not settle for someone who minimizes her accomplishments or undercuts her goals.

4. Being possessive and jealous

Research showed that although a slight amount of envy is acceptable, excessive pride is not. A self-assured lady demands autonomy and trust from her partner. Fundamental to knowing how to be a self-assured adult woman is that she won't put up with a partner who consistently questions her, limits her interactions, or invades her privacy without cause.

5. Insufficient correspondence.

A happy connection is based on strong interaction. A self-assured lady seeks a companion who shares her emotions, talks about problems in a composed manner, and listens intently. A confident woman won't put up with any of these things, therefore she has no time for vague messages, silent treatments, or avoiding crucial conversations.

6. Inequalities

In a relationship, equality extends to decision-making, tasks, and emotional investment. A self-assured woman anticipates sharing rather than taking on all of the duties and decisions. Her desire for an ideal match in which both genders contribute fairly and encourage one another is evidence of her faith in women.

7. Unfaithfulness

It is not optional to be faithful. A self-assured lady cherishes commitment and anticipates her spouse feeling the same way. In a committed marriage, infidelity defines the boundaries of what an optimistic woman is willing to and will not accept. It betrays a lack of honour and a breach of trust.

8. Gaslighting

To maintain the bar for what constitutes a mature, positive woman, a confident woman will not put up with someone who consistently tries to twist her perceptions of reality to hide their transgressions or failings.

9. Insufficient effort

Both sides must continually put work and care into their relationships. A self-assured woman is prepared to work hard and anticipates her partner doing the same. Since reciprocal effort is essential to the things a self-assured woman won't put up with, she won't put up with one-sided efforts or an individual who treats her for granted.

10. Disregarding boundaries

Creating and upholding individual limits is vital for everyone's health, and studies have shown that doing so can also strengthen marriages. A woman who exudes confidence expresses her boundaries clearly and concisely and demands that they be honoured, be they related to her privacy, her alone time, or other areas of her life.

12. Negativity

A self-assured lady seeks to create a positive, growth-oriented relationship and a life. While obstacles can occur, she is aware that persistent negativity, unjustified criticism, and pessimism can sap the happiness and love in a partnership, highlighting the significance of positivity in becoming a self-assured, mature woman.

13. The absence of emotion

In a meaningful relationship, emotional chemistry is essential. A self-assured woman looks for a companion who is empathetic, willing to listen to her feelings, and able to provide emotional support.

She is a living example of what it means to be a confident woman; she demonstrates the boundaries of what a strong woman will and will not tolerate, never settling for someone cold, uninterested, or unwilling to connect deep down.

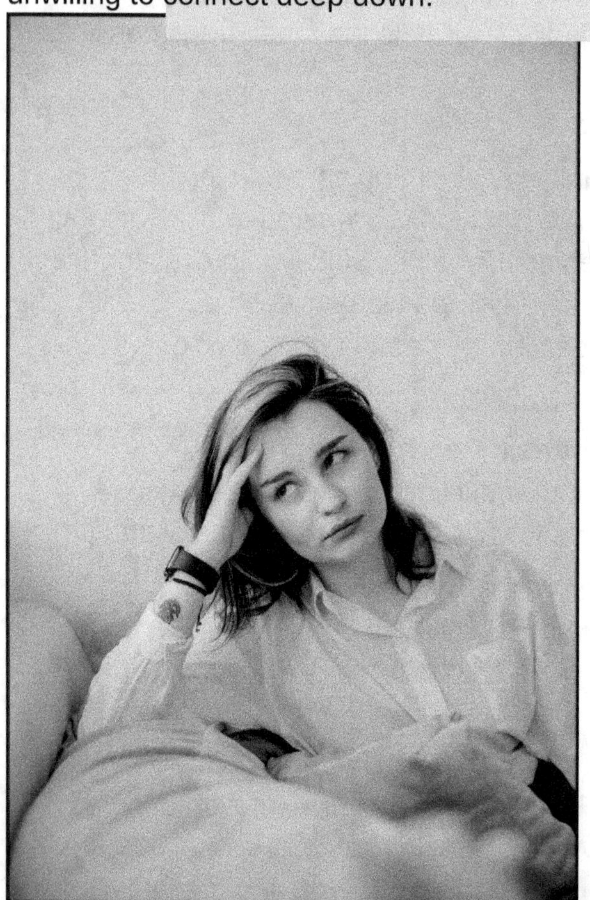

FAQs

Relationship navigation and understanding can be challenging. It's critical to distinguish between legitimate worries and high demands. This manual answers important concerns on warning signs, dialogue, judgment, and personal development to assist you in creating happier, more satisfying relationships.

How can I know whether these red flags are legitimate or if I'm just being overly picky? Determine whether your worries are about superficial characteristics or core convictions. Valid red flags usually include incompatibility with life goals, disrespect, and dishonesty.

Concerns are valid if they jeopardize your values or well-being. If not, you may be being picky by concentrating on less important preferences.

What are some constructive ways to talk to my partner about these issues?

Express your emotions using "I" phrases without placing blame on others. Engage in active listening, acknowledge and respect your partner's emotions, and schedule conversations for when you are both at ease. Transparently establish boundaries and expectations. Being open to understanding one another's viewpoints, honest, and empathetic are necessary for effective communication.

Is it preferable to let go of these red flags or should I try to mend the relationship?

Analyze how often and how severe the red flags are. Can communication and joint effort lead to their resolution? It may be healthier to let go if problems such as abuse, persistent dishonesty, or basic value conflicts are present. It could be helpful to seek professional assistance if both parties are ready to put their minds on the problems.

What are a few tips on creating self-assurance and setting firm limits in a marriage?

Determine your restrictions, requirements, and values. Be explicit by communicating the limits you set. Remind yourself of your value and take care of yourself. Remain firm and don't give in to peer pressure to cross limits. Positivity affirmations, self-awareness, and self-respect all contribute to confidence building and enhance your capacity to establish and uphold sound limits.

Last lesson learned

Essentially, the self-assured woman incorporates her respect and sense of worth into her interactions, fostering a cooperative environment based on shared ideals. She will not put up with any negative behaviour, including manipulation, rudeness, or emotional inaccessibility. These indisputably provide an atmosphere that is conducive to love, support, and development. She promotes equality and open communication while also ensuring her well-being by adhering to these norms. Her self-assurance serves as a beacon, pointing the marriage in the direction of a future marked by commitment, regard, and collaborative work in which both of you feel understood and appreciated.

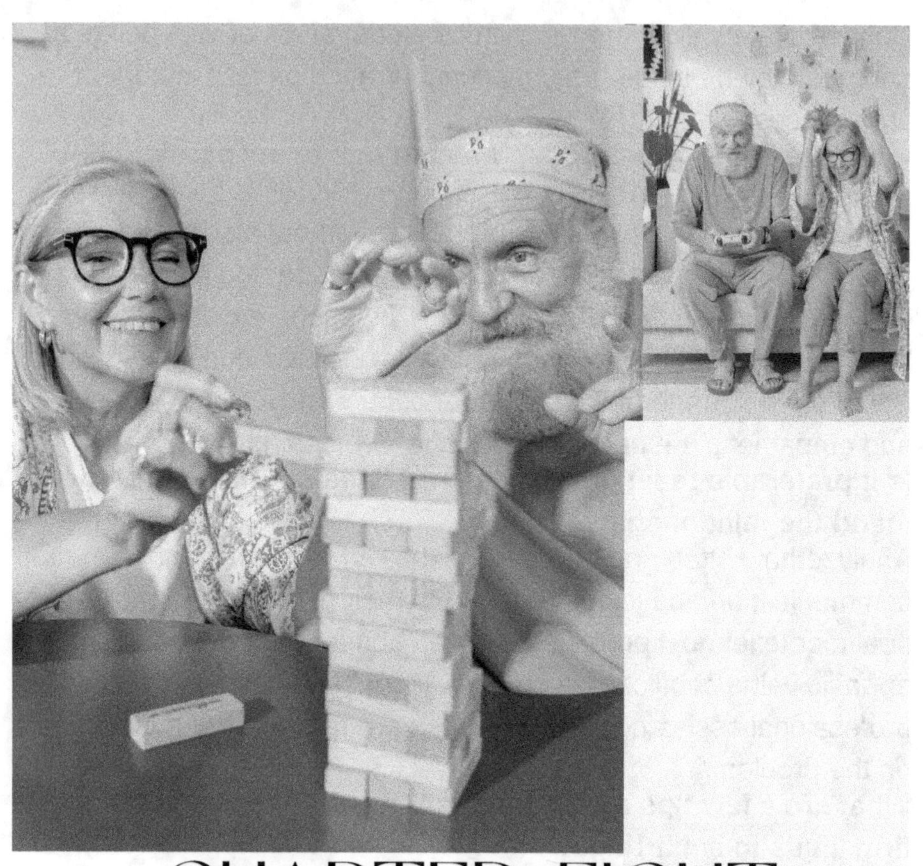

CHAPTER EIGHT

34 Imaginative Games to Light Up Your Love for Each Other.

Everything can die from a boring routine, especially your love for your family. Adding some enjoyable passionate games for lovers that are simple to learn, entertaining, and a terrific way to liven things up will help you break free from the boring routine.

Looking for entertaining games to enjoy at home or on the internet with a partner? No need to search further. To experience the enchantment for yourself, pick any of the lover's games to engage in at home. To help you ignite a flame in your marriage, try out these 35 sweet and fun fascination games built exclusively for couples!

Looking for entertaining games to enjoy at home or on the internet with a partner? No need to search further. To experience the enchantment for yourself, pick any of the lover's games to engage in at home. To help you ignite a flame in your marriage, try out these 35 sweet and fun fascination games built exclusively for couples!

How crucial is it to play games in a marriage to maintain its spark?

By bringing freshness, enjoyment, and shared knowledge into a marriage, amorous games for lovers can be extremely important for preserving the spark. Couples may bond, converse, and laugh together while playing a variety of games, whether they are card games, board games, or outdoor activities.

These times spent together create a feeling of community and serve to shake up the monotony and unleash the fun. Couples can also contribute to a more alive and satisfying marriage by engaging in love games or engaging in a fun rivalry that fosters emotional connection and a good atmosphere.

Playing games as a couple has five advantages.

There are several advantages to playing games together as a couple, including increased closeness, interaction and enjoyment.

Through shared objectives and unforgettable experiences, games improve relationships in a variety of ways, from stress reduction to the encouragement of playfulness.

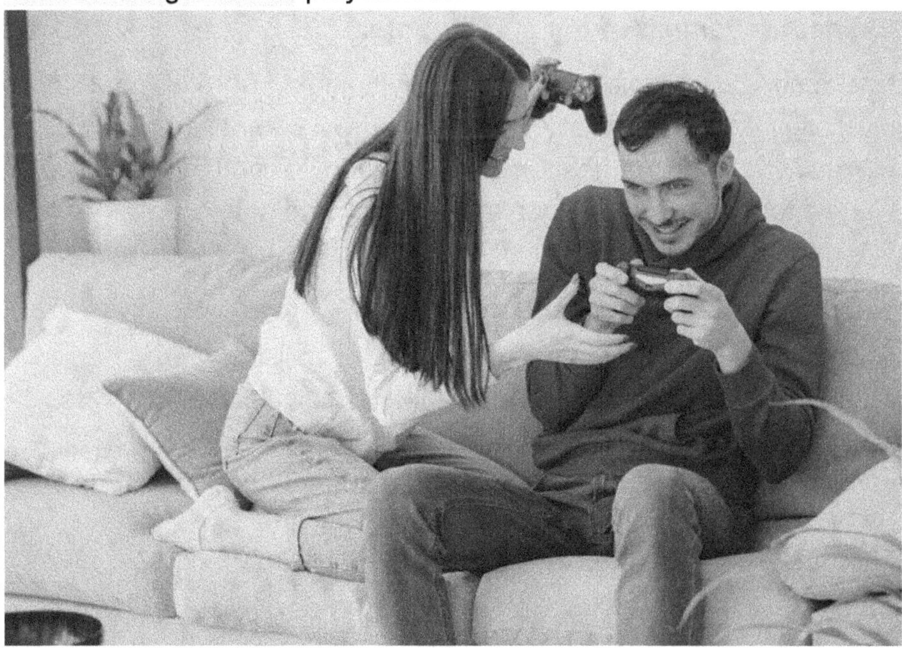

We go into more detail about a few of these advantages below:

1. Strengthening and linking

The emotional connection between spouses is reinforced when they play games together. Memorable moments are created via shared experiences, giggles, and pleasure, which strengthens bonds between people.

2. Better interaction

Strategy, cooperation, and communication are frequently needed in games. Taking part in these activities encourages couples to communicate effectively, comprehend one another's viewpoints, and cooperate to accomplish mutual goals.

3. Calming and repose

Playing games can help you relax and release tension in a fun way. Playing video games together can provide a pleasant and soothing way for couples to chill out and enjoy quality time together by taking their minds off of the worries of life daily.

4. Encouragement of joy and laughter

In a marriage, games promote creativity and an aura of fun. Play brings joy and diversity to any activity—be it competing board games, electronic games, or outdoor pursuits—and infuses positive vibes into a marriage. a couple enjoying some music.

5. Common objectives and successes

A lot of games require you to set and accomplish goals. When a couple wins a board game or conquers a difficult level in a video game, they feel a sense of satisfaction together. This mutual success increases cooperation and an aura of accomplishment, which improves the dynamic of the relationship.

34 sweet games for paired players. Taking a trip to nurture your bond and make enduring memories?

Examine these entertaining couples games which are meant to bring happiness closeness and a little bit of daring into your union. These games which range from conventional card games to creative date-night suggestions are intended to increase intimacy and promote laughing honour, and special magic that exists between you and the one you love.

This varied list ensures a moment together will be satisfying and unforgettable whether you're searching for outdoor activities or an intimate evening. Couples activities for a gathering these few games will make you and your pals giggle so check them out for the party.

1. Compose poems for one another.
Poetry is the most concrete approach to establishing a connection with your lover. Write a dirty love poem instead of something romantic. Try writing a love poem that expresses your feelings from the bottom of your heart if you want to dedicate a heartfelt expression of your feelings.

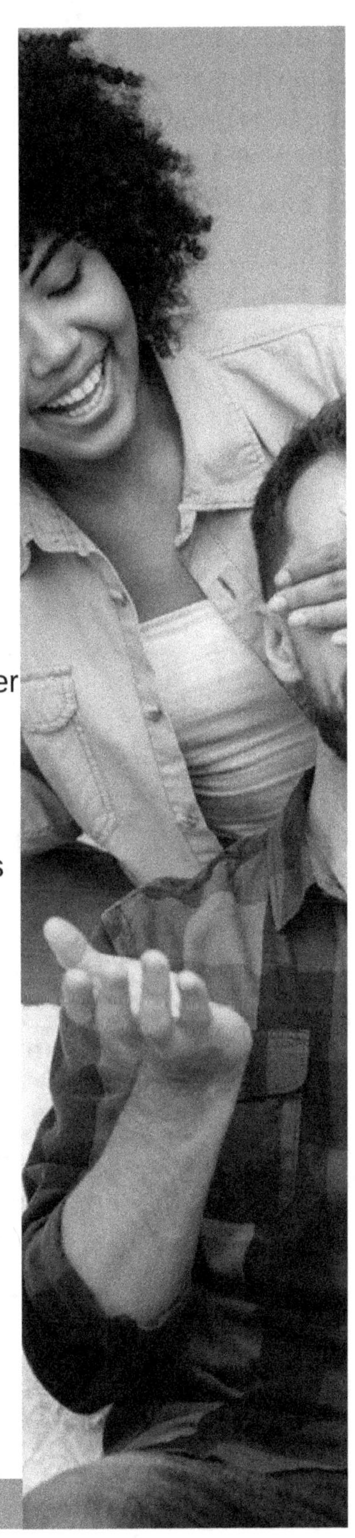

Choose your category in advance and the winner will be the one who writes the most romantic, corny, or naughty poem. a couple on the balcony conversing while sitting Poems by well-known poets might also be read aloud to your significant other.

2. Yes, No, Maybe.

In this exploratory game for girls and boys, they take turns acting as the giver and the recipient. Before beginning any of the carefully planned course of action, the donor gets the recipient's consent. If the answer is in the affirmative, the giver executes the action once.

If the recipient declines, the provider is unable to carry out the task. If the recipient responds with "maybe," the giver needs to persuade them to proceed with the deed. The provider may proceed with the activity if the recipient yields to the persuasiveness. One of the best couple games to improve your chemistry, it's the ideal tease.

3. Dare or truth

Nothing beats a game of Truth or Dare. But did you know that you could make it into one of the most entertaining, no-frills games for partners to engage in? Play it as one of a couple's favourite games with your sweetie instead of worrying about playing it with a group of pals. If they select truth, you can probe them personally or with a lighthearted inquiry; if they select dare, things will get heated.

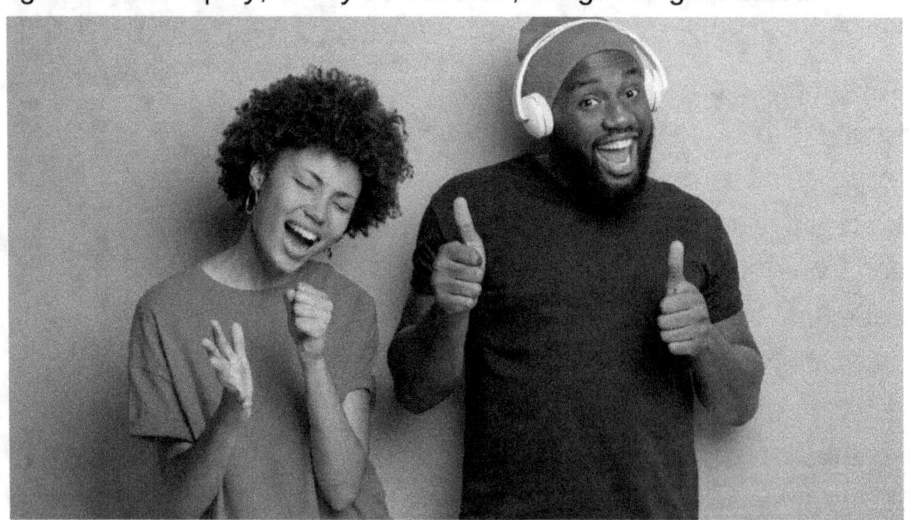

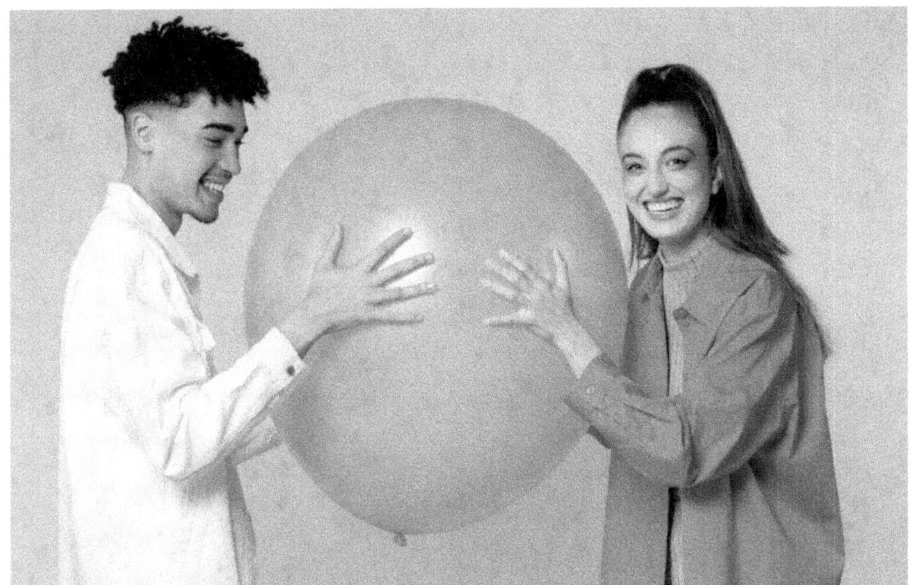

4. A bargain or no arrangement

You can elevate the concept of deal or no deal to an entirely new romantic level in your collection of pair games. With a slight modification, this standard game can become one of the most exciting and enjoyable games for couples. Simply place an envelope containing cash and a romantic wish toward your significant other, then let them make the decision.

5. Darts with balloons

Fill the surface with air balloons to kick off the competition, and then it is a turn for each pair to strike the balloon using a dart. You can maintain a few number-designated balloons scattered throughout, each with an incentive.

As an alternative, you might place the goal atop the balloon in the middle, whereupon each pair would aim. Activities with objects for couples Take a glance at these straightforward, reasonably priced, and extremely enjoyable balloon games designed for couples.

6. Release the balloon

There will be an alarm set, and the game "Blow the balloon" is uncomplicated. All of you will get a set of balloons. The competitor who blows the largest balloon during a set amount of time—let's say one minute—wins the game.

7. Burst the balloon

The balloon-blow exercise can be performed alone or as a follow-up. A lot of balloons and sharp pins are required. The winner of this game is whoever it is who bursts the greatest number of balloons in, say, a minute. As an alternative, the person who won is the one who blows out X balloons in the fastest period.

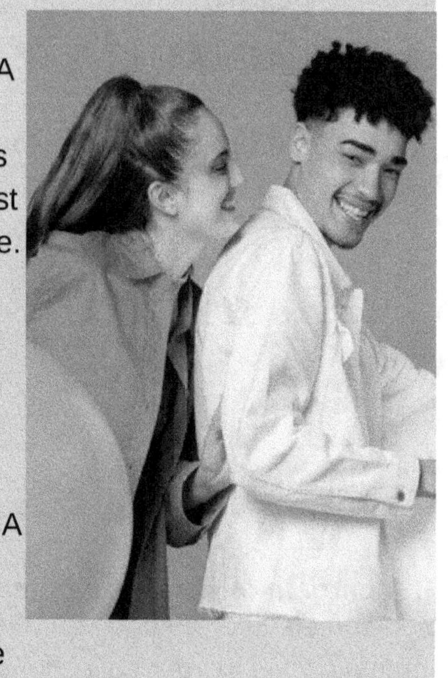

8. Roughly chop the balloon

This is a game that can be performed in groups or by couples. A razor and shaving cream are required here. In this game, your goal is to use the razor to shave the balloon without breaking it. The exciting aspect is that shaving cream will fly everywhere if the balloon busts. So be ready for that.

9. Word search balloon

There are plenty of balloons in the center of the room for this game. It is necessary to write the letters W-I-N-N-E-R on distinct balloons. The partners must compete to locate the balloons with every letter. The winner is the first person to locate the letters.

10. Use your significant other to decorate the space.

Everything is "workable," whether your lover wants a sports-themed room or you want to design a space for calmly withdrawing after a demanding day at work. Decorating your bedroom together is one of the most wonderful things you can do for the happiness of your relationship.

Recall that, similar to most aspects of a relationship, bedroom décor necessitates compromise and taking into account one another's preferences.

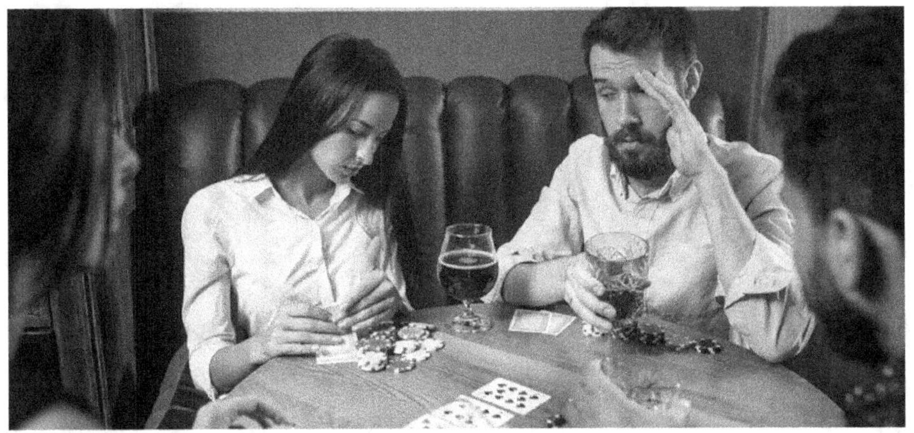

11. Tik toc amorous

You probably never would have guessed that playing tic tac toe would be included in the roster of activities for lovers. We played tic tac toe in a very simple way when we were little. It can be changed to a more amorous couple's activity.

Using sheets of paper, create cards and fill in some personal activities on them. Take another sheet of paper, make some containers and then pen several actions, like kissing, etc. Performing tic tac toe requires you to pick a position, perform the task at hand, and then continue to the next person's turn. Any request can be made of their partner by the winner of a round!

12. Poker

Do you and someone you love enjoy playing card games together? Then playing gaming is a great activity and a great game for lovers. Engage in mental challenges with one another. Let the trickery and full-time stakes begin. Make your companion take action exciting and wild by placing different bets.

13. Talk-flirt-dare

Each of you takes out a card in this card game for both partners. There are three phases to the game: daring, flirting, and conversing. To bond and participate in the game, the pair must begin with the "discussion cards." They should then play the "mingle card" to develop a closer bond and have flirty chats. Thirdly, they ought to show some audacious deeds by using the "dare cards."

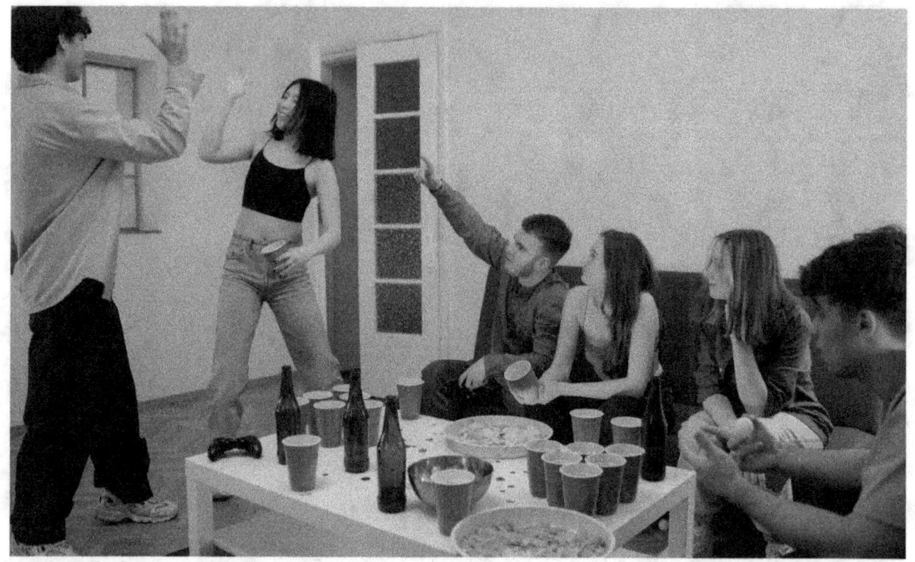

14. Drink or tell the truth

You two will get tipsy when playing this game. You will be taking out cards in this card game and challenging each other with bold questions. Playing the game encourages partners to tell the truth. They'll have to accept the drink if not.

15. A few subjects for tables

This is a game for two that aims to foster meaningful dialogue. You two can have more meaningful conversations by coming up with a few table themes. Using some wine and relaxing music, the two of you can try this game. queries for lovers to play Lovers can think deeply and speak freely with each other by playing these couples' question games.

16. Programme for excavation

Are you interested in playing quiz games with couples? Here is a fun game of questions for couples to play after that. It would be a good idea for you to ask each other intriguing and vital details about your lives rather than just the same old generic questions.

You could inquire about your partner's worst fear, covert suspicions, priceless moments, awful recollections, moments that changed their life forever, or their ideal day. Include information on your first dining experience, such as the place you dined at and the outfit you were wearing.

17. Discussion starters

Icebreaker inquiries serve as helpful instruments to start discussions to enhance partner familiarity. This is useful if the couple struggles to communicate or gets into arguments.

18. Knowledge

Trivia is a lighthearted inquiry game with questions from many genres; it doesn't focus exclusively on inquiries regarding relationships or love. You can test your partner's knowledge by asking them questions from either the entertainment or intellectual areas.

19. 21 Queries

The pairs take turns asking one another queries in 21 queries. It is possible to toggle up the query's order or ask them one after the other. When every party is requesting all 21 questions, the game is over.

20. That or this In this game,

the person asking the questions has to select one of the two possibilities that are in front of them. They are required to select one of the two options. There is no time for thought during this exciting, fast-paced questioning session, and the game can reveal any person's inclinations or motives.

Here are a few of the questions in this game: - Coffee or tea? - Nation or city? - What time is it sunrise or sunset? Dogs or cats? Beaches or hills? romantic video games These romantic couple games are likely to light up a romantic flame in your relationship.

21. Massage under blindfold

One of the hot games to play together is this one. Put on a blindfold and give your partner a massage with your hands or a certain body part. Challenge your partner to guess which body part you used. As they try to figure out which part you are using to calm their raw nerves, the guesses will get entertaining.

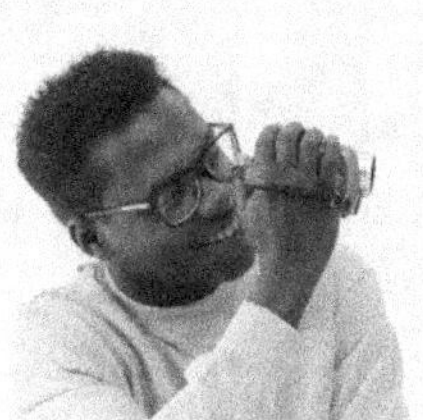

22. Love-themed Scrabble

One of the several games that everyone knows about and has played at least once in their lives is Scrabble. Have you, nonetheless, ever romantically performed this? You can spend hours, even days, playing Scrabble. You can choose!) and create guidelines dictating that you must use a word and construct a sentimental statement (that you created in Scrabble).

To one of these romantic games for couples, you can also add extra fun. It can become one of the most enjoyable games for couples to play by selecting a category like Kiss Scrabble or Strip Scrabble. Your spouse must either kiss you or take off an item of clothing after you reach a certain number of points, preferably 40 or 50. It is without a doubt one of the most well-liked love games and is a must-try for couples looking to spice things up.

23. A romantic treasure hunt

Recall Treasure Hunt! Why not make it into one of the most thrilling and enjoyable activities for couples by doing it romantically? To lead your significant other toward the last wonderful gift you have prepared for them, leave some endearing remarks. You are their favourite person (you!) or their favourite dress, or a romantic candlelight supper. Anything goes as a gift.

24. A sight

For couples looking to intensify their desire for one another, it's a delightful game. You have to look each other in the eyes to see who will look away first in this game.

If you're a couple trying to bring back the love and closeness in their marriage after a long marriage, this is a great game to play. The first spouse to turn away must take the fallout. Make the penalty enjoyable. You could request that your significant other remove a garment, give you a passionate kiss, or make you a decadent chocolate cake.

25. You have my love because

Are you looking for love games that can make you feel like an uncontrollable romantic? For lovers that are all about mush, this is the game.

22. Love-themed Scrabble

One game that the couple plays together at home is this one, which is also a terrific leveller for long-term partners.
Tell each other, one by one, why you are in love. For instance, "I love you because you make me feel my best self," "I love you because you make the best coffee for me to start the day," or "I love you because you are my biggest fanboy." The most charming games of skill for lovers Take a look at these creative games for boards that are perfect for a long-term romantic relationship.

26. A game of Scrabble

This task will test your vocabulary and spelling. In the timeless board game Scrabble, you start with seven tiles. When there are fewer tiles available, each partner gradually takes more tiles from the remainder. Placing the final letter before the other party is the major goal.

27. Monopoly

Another timeless game that takes a lot of time to play is this one. You have to own more homes than your partner to win this game. The concept is that the other party will have to pay higher rent for the land in your space the more properties you own.

28. Parcheesi

The rules of Parcheesi are as follows: the players take a seat on the other side and arrange their colours in a big circle to their right. Instead of rolling the dice all at once, the players divide up their actions according to the number on the dice. The first person to get all four pieces inside the house wins.

29. Chess

Without an introduction, chess ranks as one of many well-known and ancient games. The black and white pieces must first be arranged neatly in sequence. There are specific movements for every piece on the board. This video will teach you how to play the game if you're a novice:

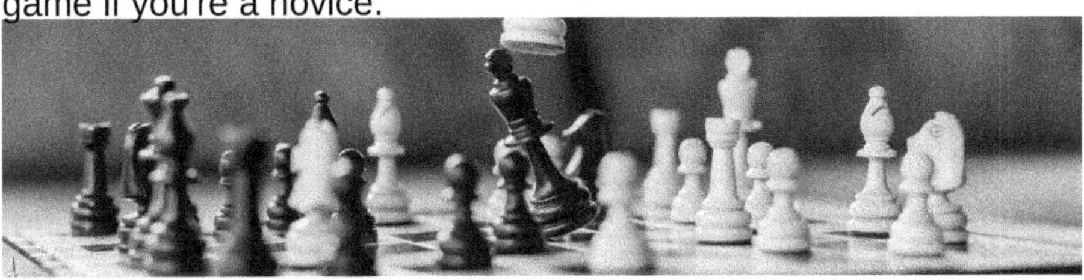

30. Hive

It is a classic game that is comparable to this one. Each piece moves in a particular way in this game as well. The objective of this two-player game is to encircle the opposing party's queen with your insect pieces. wholesome games for couples Play these enjoyable activities that will be enjoyable for married couples together. Have fun!

32. The image gaming

Creating your own game rules is not a bad idea. You can take part in all the fun by creating your own couple's game. You can take a little box and use picture paste to decorate it whatever you like. Throw the box-shaped dice now, and your partner must comply with the image's instructions. You can use images of couples kissing, etc.

33. A ripoff film

It can be enjoyable to see a movie together. Why not give it a little spiciness and make it one of the most entertaining games that couples can play at home? Play a romantic comedy and don't be afraid to act out the scenarios with your significant other. It might add some excitement to your boring foreplay sessions.

34. Paint a canvas of love upon each other's bodies.

Go crazy in the bedroom and express yourself freely about each other's bodies. Place a mat that can be washed. Use playpens, chocolate syrup, whipped cream, or edible body paint to decorate each other's bodies. Go to the bathroom and take turns bathing each other with a luxurious shower gel. It's also one of the most sexy games to play foreplay with your partner. These kinds of relationship games are a terrific method to foster greater communication between spouses.

Attempt these enjoyable and charming activities for lovers, and see which of them you and your lover end up like the most. These couple's games are guaranteed to help you two reconnect with one another.

35. Allow the ship to sink
One of the famous and entertaining games for adults is Sink the Ship, but you can play it romantically to make it one of the greatest games for couples. Invite a friend to join you in the game, and if you lose, you must do anything your opponent demands of you. Play this love game and let your thoughts run wild.

A Frequently Asked Questions
It is a lovely adventure to improve your relationship through games. These tips for creating happiness and closeness cover everything from frequency to game choice.

What frequency of gaming should a couple engage in?
Continual participation is essential. When it comes to regular opportunities for interaction, strike a balance that works for both of you, whether it's impromptu gaming dates or a weekly board game night.

Which games are best for your relationship, and how can you choose them?
Choose cooperative or competitive games according to your preferences and those that foster common interests or communication. Continuity keeps things interesting.

How do we make romantic games that we own?
Incorporate shared memories, add personal touches, and customize rules to suit your needs. Tailor-made games provide unforgettable experiences and strengthen bonds between players.

Playing games made especially for couples is indispensable.
These games frequently address relational issues, however they are not necessary. To create a customized experience that appeals to both partners, modify popular games or design unique activities.

Key Observation
These games for husbands and wives are ideal for spending quality time together at home, as they will strengthen your bond and make your time together enjoyable. For some relaxing time, give these a try!

Chapter Nine
50+ Marital sayings suitable for all lovers

With these marriage-related quotes and messages for the love of your existence, you can immerse yourself in the romanticism of the present marriage or your upcoming nuptials. For as long as people have been able to write, people have written about love, which is a multifaceted concept.

These fifty marriage-related quotations will encourage you to commit and will effectively communicate your feelings to your spouse. Use these sayings as the caption for your Valentine's Day cards, thank-you cards, wedding announcements, and social media pictures of you and your partner.

Marriage sayings suitable for all couples

These happy marriage quotes, long marriage quotes, and quotes for newly married couples should offer you some perspective on your lucky relationship, regardless of your goals for it—longevity, contentment, or tax breaks.

1. "If I marry, I want to marry well."
2. "Many falls in love, always with the same person, are necessary for a successful marriage." 3. "Forgetting your wife's birthday is the most wonderful way to remember it once."
4. "The finest present you can give someone is your time."
5. "I adore having a spouse. Finding that one special someone you want to irritate for every moment of your life is such a terrific feeling."
6. "When you can go grocery shopping together, you know you're in love."

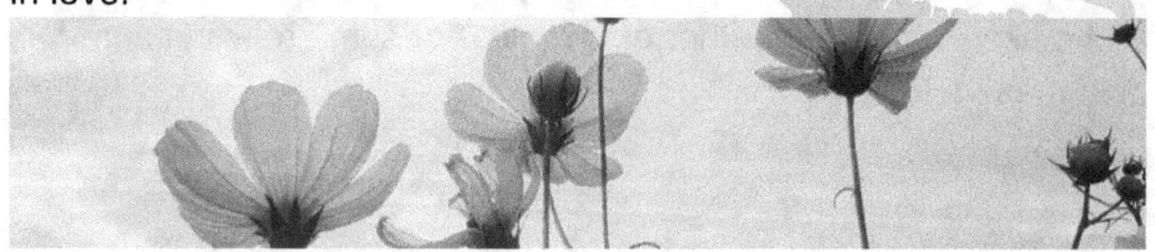

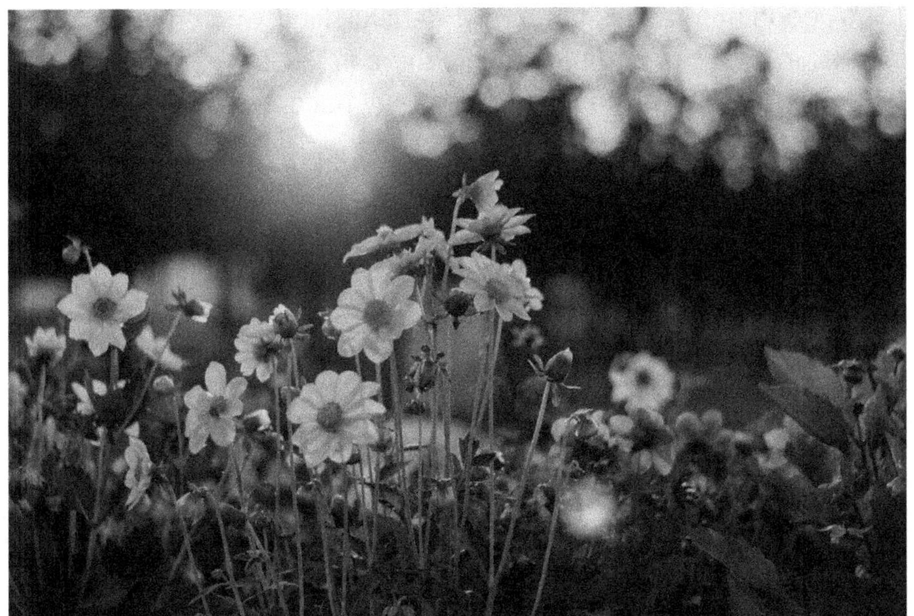

7. "My ability to convince my wife to marry me was my most outstanding accomplishment."
8. "You should have someone use a computer with slow internet before you marry them so you can get to know them better."
9. "Is there anything more significant for two human beings than to experience a sense of eternal union – supporting one another during every challenge, finding solace in one another's grief, and providing silent, indescribable recollections during their final moments together?"
10. "Love must be made, like bread; it must be constantly remade and made new; it does not simply sit there, like a stone."
11. "Let there be gaps in your closeness and let the breezes of the heavens flow between you,"
12. "Love each other, but don't let your love become a bond; instead, let it flow like an ocean between the coastline of your hearts."
13. "Being together as the 'ideal pair' is not the recipe for an outstanding marriage." It occurs when a flawed pair discovers joy in their uniqueness."

14. "A good marriage is the most beautiful, kind, and endearing friendship, unity, or companionship there is."

15. "It's easy to grasp love at first sight; it becomes a miracle when two people look at each other for a lifetime."

16. "A fulfilling marriage is a lengthy conversation that never seems to end." The key to a happy union is matching with the correct partner. If all you want to do is be with them, then you know they're right.

17. "Marriage is the greatest source of happiness on earth."

18. Come on, let's take care of each other and be a cosy couple! We will be very happy to have someone we can chat to and spend time with no matter what."

19. "A healthy marriage permits personal development and evolution in both lovers as well as in their modes of expressing love."

20. The strongest marriages are based on cooperation. A good dosage of adoration, a boundless supply of elegance affection, and kindness.

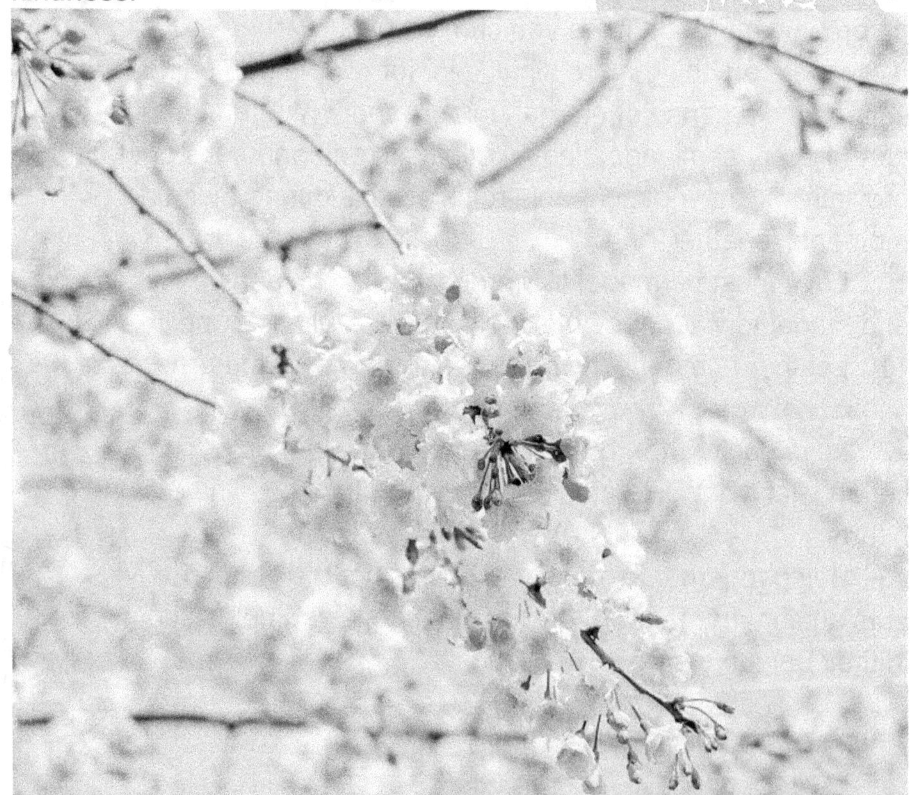

It's simple to become overloaded by the many aspects of your weddings, so take a moment to go over these wedding sayings for newlyweds embarking on their journey. Moreover, you may use these pearls of wisdom to spice up your big-day invitations, congratulate friends who have recently gotten married, or pen comments for pictures in an album for a wedding.

1. "You are interested in every moment of your life to begin as soon as you decide you would like to share it with someone for the rest of your days."

2. "Upon Harry's Meeting Sally Consider this before getting married: Do you think you can have a meaningful conversation with your spouse far into old age? All other aspects of marriage are ephemeral."

3. "Never get married to a man you wouldn't want to split up with."

4. "The true act of marriage happens in the heart, not in the church, synagogue, or ballroom. It's a decision you make, and how you treat your spouse reflects that decision. Not only on your wedding day but many times after."

5. "May the happiness of the bride and groom shine like the light of the morning, and their sorrows be mere shadows that disappear in the sunlight of love."

6. "Don't assume that just because you're married, the romance is over."

7. "Happy marriages grow when we love the people we marry, and they start when we marry the people we love."

8. "When wonderful people get together, as they usually do, it is such a happiness."

9. "Grow old with me, for the best is still to come."

10. "I love you for who you are, and for who I become when we are together. I adore you for who you are becoming and not just for what you have been."

11. "When two hearts are in love, words cannot express their feelings."
12. Marcelime An anniversary of marriage is a celebration of tolerance, perseverance, love, and trust. The sequence is different for every year."
Quotations about romance and love

Quotations about romance and love

Do you have a strong romantic interest but aren't quite ready to commit? Take some inspiration from these romantic quotations and present them to the person you love on Valentine's Day itself, your anniversary, or every other fundamental celebration.
1. "Life exists where love exists."
2. "To be loved in any case and to be truly seen by somebody then is a human sacrifice that can almost seem magical."
3. "When you can't sleep because reality finally surpasses your dreams, you know you're in love."
4. "Love has no boundaries. It goes over walls, over fences, and over barriers to reach its target with hope."
5. "To experience love and love-making is to feel the sun shining on all sides."
6. "I could spend forever strolling around my garden if I had a flower for every time I thought about you."
7. "You gain courage when you love someone deeply, and you gain strength when someone loves you deeply."
8. "You want someone who will take the bus with you when the limo breaks down, but a lot of people want to ride with you in the limo."
9. "Being dumb together is love."
10. "Each of us is a little strange. Life is also a little strange. We join forces with someone whose weirdness aligns with our own, fall into mutually pleasurable craziness, and refer to this state of affairs as real love."

11. "It's simple to get back up after falling in love. However, once you fall in love, it's tough to stop."

12. "Keep in mind that even when you're too sluggish to say it yourself, sending the best Valentine's Day card demonstrates your concern and thoughtfulness."

13. "Valentine's Day alone makes February seem like, well, January.

14. "Love is like a lovely flower that I may never touch, yet even without touching it, its smell fills the garden with joy."

15. "What we loved was more than just love."

16. "Every heart begins to sing, imperfectly, until another heart begins to mumble in response. There is always a song for those who want to sing. Everyone can become a poet at the touch of a lover."

17. "Is there anyone who is impoverished and loves?"

18. "What does love entail? I once came upon a very impoverished young man who was in love on the streets. A waterlogged shoe, a worn-out coat, an ancient cap, and stars in his soul all came together."

19. "You grinned because you knew that I fell in love the moment I saw you."

20. "The only way to heal love is to love more."

21. "Love is the one word that lifts all the burdens and suffering from life."

22. "Live by love even though the stars walk backwards. Trust your heart if the seas catch fire." For example, cummings.

CHAPTER TEN

Two Keys for a Joyful Marriage.

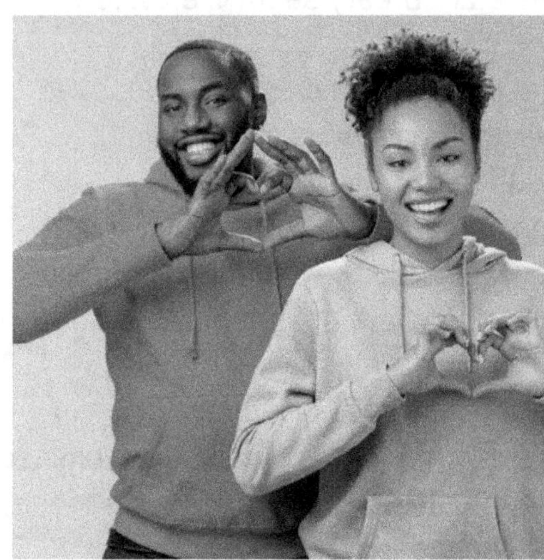

Nearly all marriages begin with a lavish ceremony. Every couple, together with their loved ones, has high expectations for their future together. However, achieving marital happiness is not a simple task. And many couples choose not to finish the voyage, as the all too familiar divorce rates of today show.

It would be simple to place the blame for our high divorce rate on things like failing to maintain open lines of communication, letting resentment and bitterness fester in our hearts, and not spending enough quality time together. Books, articles, and seminars abound that offer advice on how to enhance these and a host of other relationship-related topics. However, even while spending quality time together, forgiving one another, and communicating are essential to a happy marriage, their absence is typically an indication of a far more serious issue. Furthermore, no amount of external behaviour adjustment will be effective until this issue is resolved.

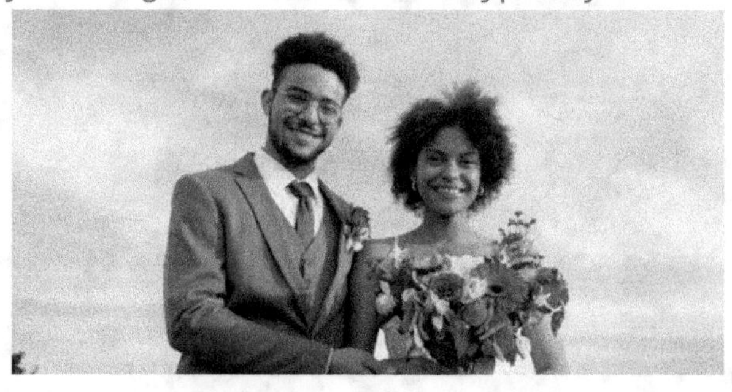

Let's examine the following verse from the Bible to get a sense of what this more profound problem might be: "Teacher, which is the most important rule in the Law?" asked one them, a legal expert, to put Jesus to the test. Jesus answered back: "With all of your brain, spirit, and heart, you need to love your Creator, your heavenly Father.

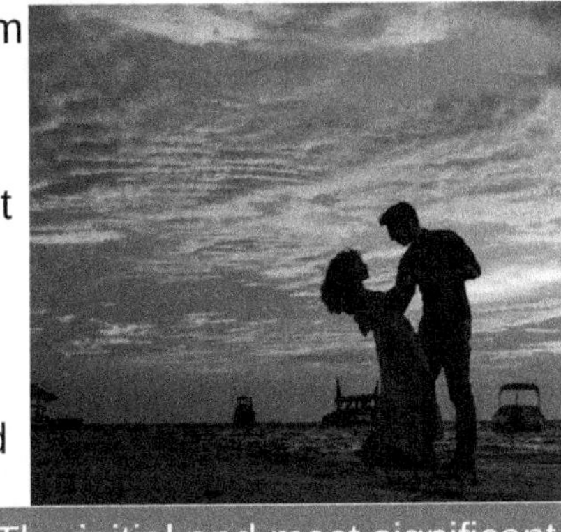

The initial and most significant commandment is this one. And it's similar to the second: "Treat other people with respect." These two laws are the cornerstone of all legal principles and those of the prophets.
Matthew 22:35–40 I think that breaking one of these two laws by one or both partners is the root cause of almost every marriage issue. This holds for any kind of relationship. Trouble is inevitable the moment we start prioritizing our needs and desires over those of God or our significant other.

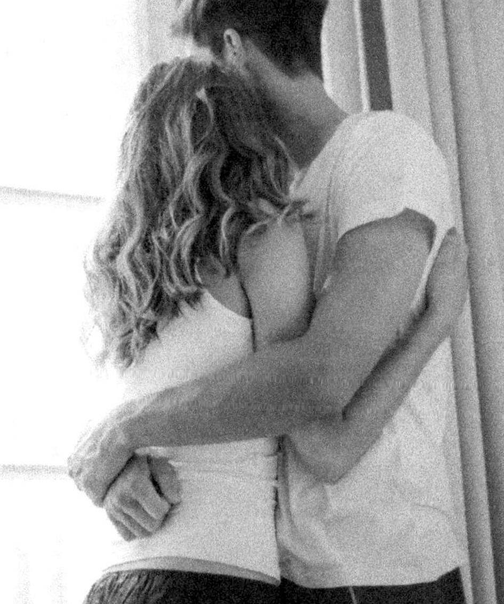

Are you having issues communicating in your marriage?

At what rate do you listen to God or your partner instead of demanding more time on the air? Are you beginning to feel hatred and animosity toward your partner?

When was the most recent time you genuinely praised God for his blessing with them and brought them before you in prayer? Have trouble getting together for quality time? Consider asking God in a prayer with your significant other how he wants you to spend your time.

You'll notice that as soon as you start doing these things, your attention naturally starts to move from God and your spouse to yourself and your desires. As a result, you undoubtedly desire to spend more time together, communication issues start to get better, and anger and resentment start to vanish. Naturally, you can't count on such improvements to materialize quickly.

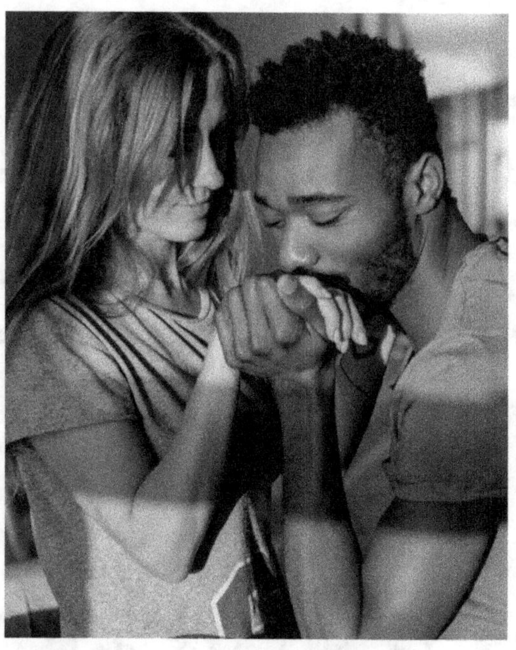

Financial strains, parenting concerns, and other uncontrollable obstacles may inevitably arise in your partnership. However, your union will be resilient to any adversity if you dedicate your union to God and consciously choose to prioritize God and your spouse every day. Furthermore, you'll enjoy a ton of exciting activities with each other throughout the route!

Have you had trouble keeping your spouse happy in your marriage?

Maybe it's time for you and your partner to ask God to guide your union. We invite you to pray the following if you so choose: "Dear God, I am so grateful that you brought us together to be a pair. We ask you, Lord Jesus, to pardon our past self-centeredness and enter our lives and marriage.

Please provide us with the ability to prioritize You and one another every day. Make others benefit from our partnership. Above all, let it be a blessing for You. Amen."

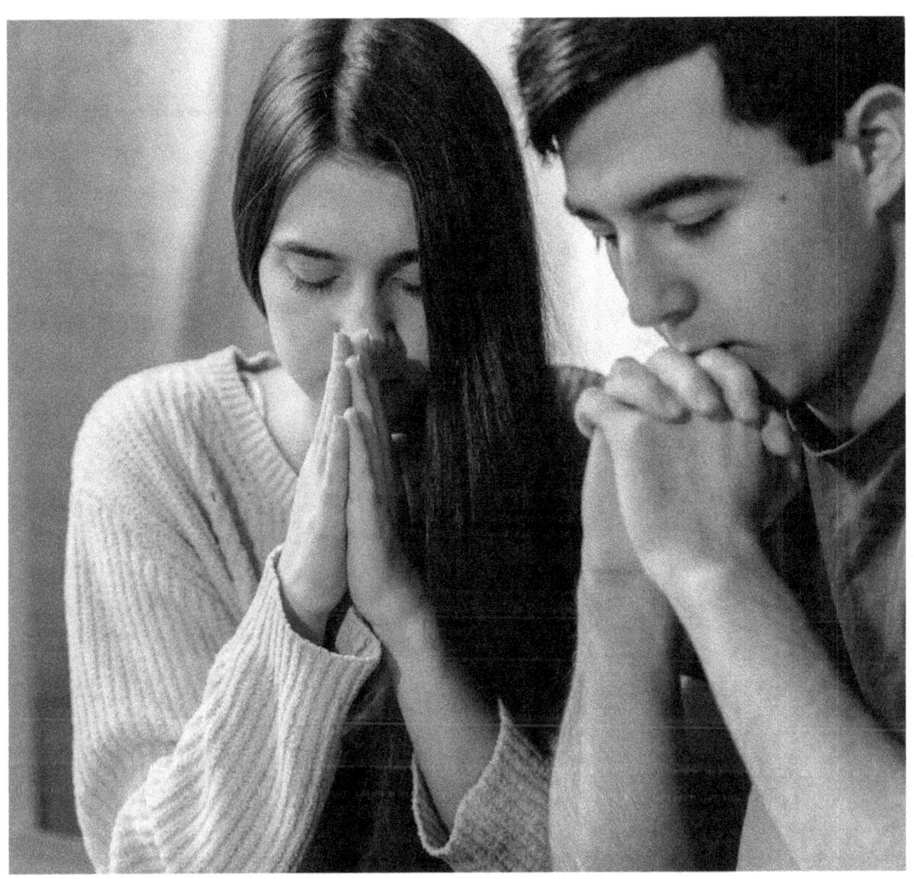

Prayer is the master key, connecting with God and boosting your spirituality is a must-do activity for couples

Conclusion

Matrimony is an exciting trip. A wonderful marriage doesn't just happen. Instead, you learn about it day by day. At times, it feels exhilarating! At other times, it's a taxing ascent. Since life happens, no one can plot out their union in its entirety.

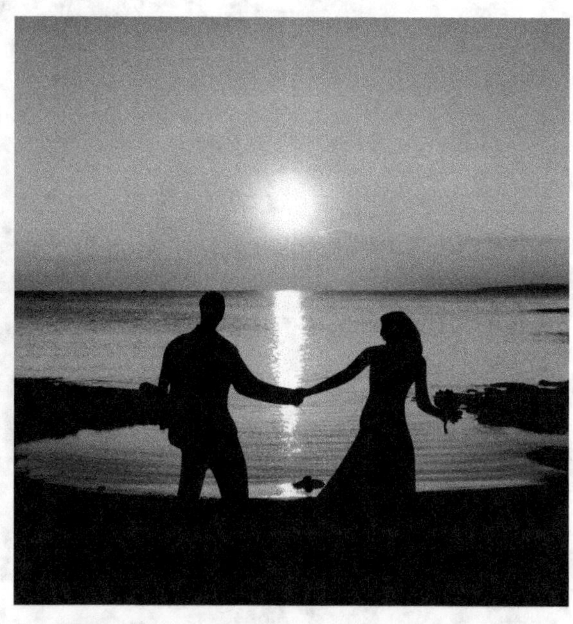

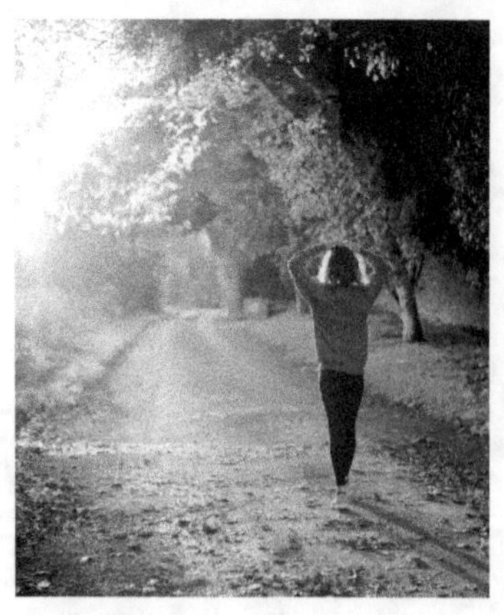

However, as you walk through the years shared, you'll discover things you may undertake to ensure your partnership is prepared for anything that reaches up. Below are some words of wisdom from experts to help you on your way toward matrimony.

Create a unique bond.

Choose an item that best captures how you interact and turn it into your own. It might be as easy as getting together on a regular Friday morning for tea and talk or playing card games on the following day. Sometimes you enjoy watching concerts on Netflix and schedule time every week to listen to songs together.
That is customary. And by all means, feel free to laugh, dance, and sing! Your bond with one another might grow stronger and more profound through rituals. Certain couples take pleasure in public rituals, such as dressing in matching colours. Hold your laughter. That's what we would do!

The words you say matter a lot in our marital life.

Be respectful of one another both outside and inside of your home. Whether or not your lover is there, you ought to treat them with kindness whenever you speak about them in public. When it's simply the two of you, you ought to handle your partner with dignity in both your words and deeds. Respect for your partner fosters love and trust in addition to.

Pay attention to the positive

Enjoy yourself and your marital life, but remember not to take anything for granted in your union. Marriage needs to be deliberate. Even when you don't feel like it, decide to live by with each other. Philippians 4:8–9 emphasises the positive traits that make each other "great and thankworthy"! The Almighty Lord pledges to make your relationships and hearts at peace. "Whatsoever is admirable and commendable, satisfying, genuine, and just, God of peace will be with you if you consider these possessions.

You could be extremely incorrect as well as right.

Make a conscious effort to speak with one another. At least as essential as what you say is how you say it—that is, how you convey your insight and point of view through tone, timing, and delivery.

You won't get through if your communication style and timing are more crucial than the words you convey. Another interaction technique is to bear in mind that even in disagreements, you are all members of the same side with common objectives. Treat one another with respect.

Pay attention and take note of your distinctions.

We got into a heated argument about something recent in our marital life. In my own family, that was not exceptional, but in Glory's family, it was. He withdrew from the conversation since it seemed to him to be an aggressive argument. After a few moments, I can hardly remember our conversation.
The identical event may appear extremely different to you and your partner. Thus, pose inquiries. Next, pay close attention while you listen to comprehend the other person's perspective. As needed, give each other some space. However, discuss it when you're all set. Don't just ignore your emotions and go on. Make the most of these chances to strengthen your inner bond, which fosters connectivity. You and your spouse can truly benefit from differences in your family.

Have bravery of character!

Everybody makes mistakes. There will be occasions in a marriage when one or both partners make blunders, and these missteps can put a great deal of strain on the family. Forgiveness is easy for certain missteps, but it takes time to heal for others.
Making bad decisions in your marital life can occasionally land you in the "18-yard box." For a spell, you can even be "controlled to the bench."

When you feel like you're "on the bench," or cut off from your partner, what goes through your mind? Do you ever fear that the game may be too hard for you to return to? It is still promising to find happiness in your marital life, so keep this in mind before you "throw in the towel" or begin to feel like "all hope seems gone."

However, trust is necessary, and one may need to modify one's attitude. Scripture encourages us to have bravery. "Have faith in your heavenly father, and he boost your heart. Be brave." Psalm 27:14.

A focused mind is capable of bringing about modification. It sounds like optimistic reasoning, and that's exactly it. If you have a strong will, you can turn your marital life around and put it back on the road to pleasure and joy. Regaining direction is not always simple, particularly during trying times, but it is achievable with God's assistance.